CHAIR YOGA
For Seniors
TO LOSE WEIGHT

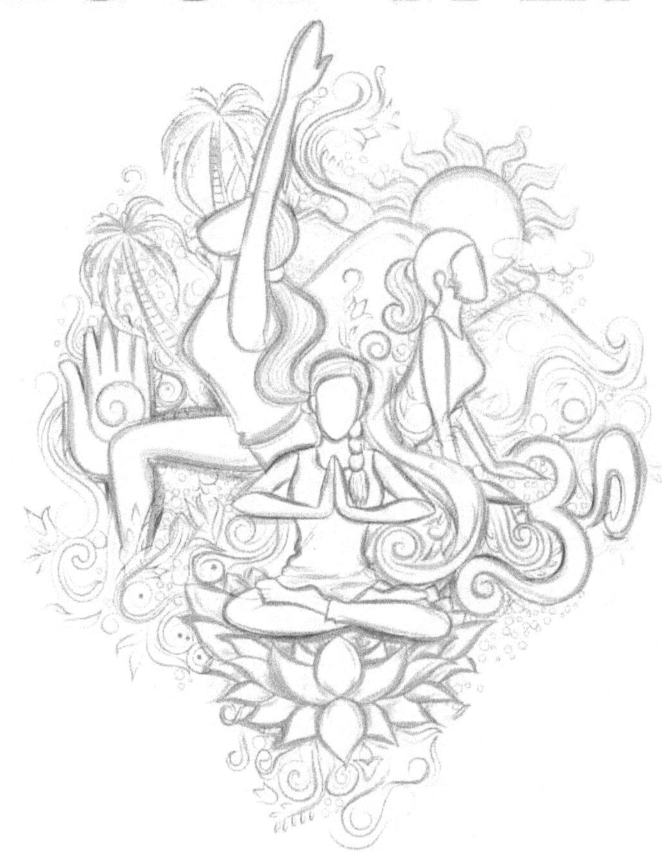

LOSE BELLY FAT WITH JUST 10 MINUTES A DAY OF LOW-IMPACT EXERCISES ALL WHILE SITTING DOWN. EMBARK ON A 28-DAY BODY REVOLUTION CHALLENGE.

HEATHER MOORE

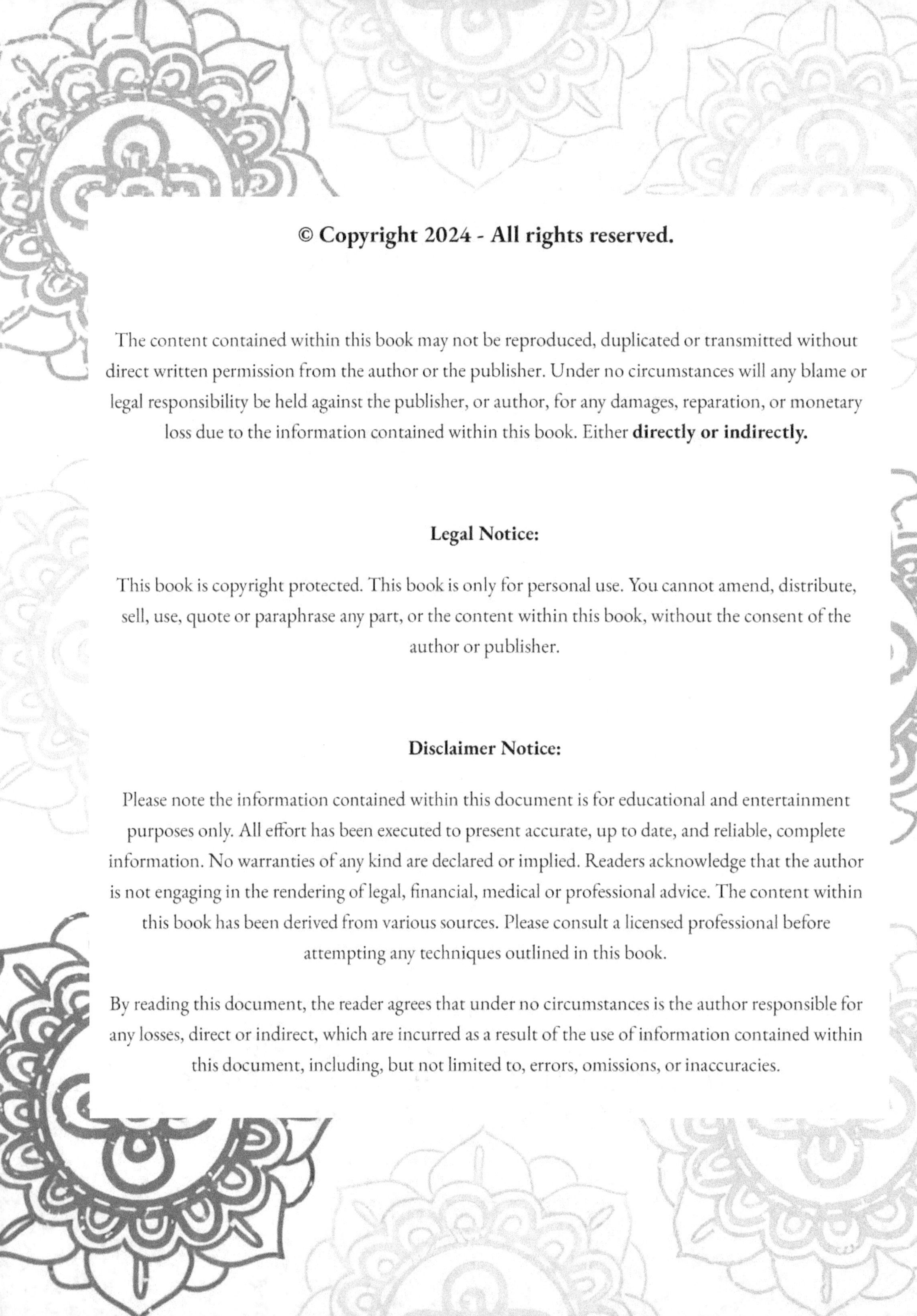

Table of Contents

INTRODUCTION

Fundamentals of Chair Yoga

Chair Yoga, as a form of yoga, is tailored to be accessible and beneficial to individuals regardless of their physical condition, age, or fitness level. By utilizing a chair either as the primary support for exercises or as an aid in balance and flexibility practices, Chair Yoga makes the wide-ranging benefits of traditional yoga practices available to those who may find standard yoga poses challenging. This adaptation not only opens up the world of yoga to a broader audience but also ensures that the practice can be safely and effectively incorporated into daily routines, contributing to overall wellness and health.

Definition of Chair Yoga

At its core, Chair Yoga is defined by the use of a chair to perform yoga poses and sequences. This innovative approach allows participants to experience the physical and mental benefits of yoga without the need to get down onto a yoga mat. The chair provides stability and support, enabling practitioners to hold poses longer and with proper alignment, which enhances the effectiveness of the practice. It is particularly suited for seniors, individuals with mobility or balance issues, those recovering from injury, or anyone who spends a significant portion of their day seated.

Essential Elements of Chair Yoga

Equipment Needed

The primary piece of equipment required for Chair Yoga is a sturdy, armless chair. This ensures that movements and poses can be performed without obstruction. The chair should be stable enough to support the practitioner's weight during various exercises. Additionally, comfortable clothing that allows for a full range of motion and a pair of non-slip shoes or bare feet to maintain stability on the floor are recommended.

Adaptation of Traditional Poses

Chair Yoga modifies traditional yoga poses to be performed while seated or using the chair for support. These adaptations ensure that the essence and benefits of the original poses are retained while making them accessible. For example, a seated forward bend can be performed to stretch the spine and shoulders, while a standing warrior pose can be adapted using the chair for balance and support.

Focus on Accessibility

One of the fundamental principles of Chair Yoga is its focus on making yoga accessible to everyone. It eliminates the need to get down on the floor, making yoga achievable for those with limited mobility or those who find traditional yoga poses too challenging. This inclusivity extends the benefits of yoga practice, such as improved flexibility, strength, and mental clarity, to a wider audience.

Benefits of Chair Yoga

Chair Yoga offers numerous physical and mental benefits. Physically, it helps increase flexibility, improve muscle tone, boost circulation, and enhance balance and coordination. The support of the chair allows individuals to safely perform stretches and strength-building exercises without the risk of strain or injury. Mentally, Chair Yoga promotes relaxation and stress reduction. The focus on breathing and mindful movement helps calm the mind, reduce anxiety, and enhance overall well-being.

Getting Started with Chair Yoga

Choosing the Right Chair

Selecting the right chair is crucial. It should be sturdy and stable without arms. The seat should not be too soft; a firm seat helps with posture during exercises. The height of the chair should allow the feet to be flat on the ground with knees at a 90-degree angle.

Creating a Safe Space

Ensure there is enough space around the chair to perform movements without obstruction. The area should be free from slip hazards, and there should be sufficient room to extend the arms and legs during various poses.

Starting with Guidance

For those new to Chair Yoga, starting with guided sessions through classes or online tutorials is advisable. This ensures that the poses are performed correctly and safely. Over time, as familiarity and comfort with the practices increase, individuals may explore creating their own sequences based on their specific needs and goals.

Conclusion

Chair Yoga stands out as a versatile and inclusive form of exercise that adapts the ancient practice of yoga to meet modern needs and limitations. Its focus on using a chair for support makes yoga accessible to a broader audience, offering a gentle yet effective way to improve physical health and mental well-being. By emphasizing safe, accessible, and adaptable practices, Chair Yoga ensures that the transformative power of yoga can be experienced by all, making it a valuable tool for enhancing quality of life.

Breathing and Meditation

Breathing and meditation, integral components of yoga, including Chair Yoga, extend beyond physical exercise to touch the realms of mental and emotional well-being. These practices, deeply rooted in ancient yoga traditions, have found a place in modern wellness routines, offering profound benefits to practitioners of all ages and physical capabilities. This section delves into the essence of breathing and meditation within the context of Chair Yoga, exploring their definitions, the minimal requirements for practice, and the myriad benefits they offer.

Understanding Breathing and Meditation

Breathing (Pranayama): In yoga, breathing exercises are referred to as Pranayama, which literally means "control of life force." Pranayama practices involve altering the speed, depth, and pattern of breathing. Through controlled breathing, practitioners can influence their physiological state, moving from states of arousal or stress to states of calm and relaxation.

Meditation: Meditation in the context of yoga is a practice of focused attention. It involves directing the mind to a single point of reference, which could be a breath, a mantra, or a specific thought. The goal of meditation is to cultivate a state of heightened awareness and inner peace, reducing the clutter of thoughts and allowing the practitioner to experience a sense of calm and clarity.

Essentials for Practicing Breathing and Meditation

Practicing breathing and meditation requires very little in terms of physical equipment. The primary requirement is a quiet, comfortable space where one can sit or recline without interruption. While Chair Yoga incorporates the use of a chair for physical exercises, it also serves as an excellent prop for seated breathing exercises and meditation. A sturdy, armless chair that allows the feet to rest flat on the floor is ideal.

For those who prefer, a yoga mat or cushion can be used for additional comfort, especially if one chooses to meditate in a seated position on the floor prior to or following their Chair Yoga routine. However, the essence of breathing and meditation practices lies not in the physical setup but in the practitioner's engagement with the process.

Benefits of Breathing and Meditation Exercises

The benefits of incorporating breathing and meditation exercises into one's daily routine, particularly within the Chair Yoga framework, are extensive, impacting both physical health and mental well-being.

Physical Health:

- **Improved Respiratory Function:** Regular practice of pranayama can enhance lung capacity and efficiency, which is particularly beneficial in increasing oxygenation and supporting overall vitality.
- **Lowered Blood Pressure:** Both breathing exercises and meditation have been shown to reduce blood pressure by calming the nervous system, offering a natural remedy for hypertension.
- **Enhanced Digestive Function:** The relaxation and stress reduction associated with these practices can improve digestive efficiency, addressing issues like bloating and irregularity.

Mental and Emotional Well-being:

- **Stress Reduction:** One of the most immediate benefits of breathing and meditation is a significant reduction in stress. These practices activate the parasympathetic nervous system, promoting relaxation and reducing cortisol levels.
- **Improved Concentration and Focus:** Regular meditation cultivates a sharper focus and better concentration by training the mind to remain present and undistracted.
- **Emotional Balance:** Engaging in these practices can lead to greater emotional resilience and stability by providing tools to manage anxiety, depression, and emotional fluctuations.

Incorporating Breathing and Meditation into Your Routine

Starting Simple: Begin with just a few minutes of breathing exercises or meditation each day, gradually increasing the duration as you become more comfortable with the practice.

Consistency is Key: The benefits of breathing and meditation are cumulative, meaning consistent practice over time yields the most significant results.

Use Guided Practices: For beginners, guided breathing exercises and meditations can provide structure and direction, helping to familiarize oneself with the techniques and their intended effects.

Integrate with Chair Yoga: Incorporate breathing exercises at the beginning of your Chair Yoga session to center and calm the mind, preparing it for physical activity. Conclude with a meditation practice to assimilate the benefits of the session, enhancing the sense of relaxation and well-being.

Conclusion

Breathing and meditation offer a pathway to profound health benefits that complement the physical practices of Chair Yoga. By integrating these practices into your daily routine, you can enhance not only your physical health through improved respiratory function and reduced blood pressure but also your mental and emotional well-being by fostering stress reduction, improved focus, and emotional balance. The simplicity and accessibility of these practices make them an invaluable addition to any wellness regimen, requiring nothing more than a willingness to engage and a few minutes of dedicated time each day.

Why Chair Yoga is Effective for Weight Loss

Chair Yoga, often perceived as a gentle form of exercise tailored primarily towards seniors or individuals with limited mobility, holds surprising potential in the realm of weight loss and metabolic health. Despite its seemingly low-impact nature, Chair Yoga effectively contributes to weight management and overall wellness through a combination of metabolic stimulation, cardiovascular conditioning, and mindful eating encouragement. This exploration delves into the mechanisms through which Chair Yoga aids in shedding excess weight, enhancing metabolic function, and promoting a healthier lifestyle.

Stimulating Metabolism Through Gentle Movement

One of the fundamental ways Chair Yoga supports weight loss is by enhancing metabolic rate. The series of movements and poses, even though performed while seated or using a chair for support, engage various muscle groups across the body. This engagement requires energy, thereby stimulating the metabolism. The metabolic boost from regular Chair Yoga practice, though perhaps more subtle than that from high-intensity workouts, is significant, especially when considering the accessibility and sustainability of the practice for individuals at different fitness levels.

- **Muscle Engagement and Maintenance:** Muscle tissue is metabolically active, meaning it burns calories even at rest. Chair Yoga helps in maintaining and even building muscle mass, which in turn supports a higher resting metabolic rate. By incorporating poses that require holding and muscle engagement, Chair Yoga ensures that practitioners are not only stretching but also subtly strengthening their bodies.

- **Improved Digestive Function:** The twists, forward bends, and stretches in Chair Yoga can aid digestive health, which is crucial for efficient metabolism. These movements help stimulate the digestive organs, promoting better nutrient absorption and more efficient waste elimination, both of which are essential for weight management.

Cardiovascular Conditioning with Chair Yoga

While Chair Yoga is generally low-impact, it can still provide cardiovascular benefits, especially for those who might not be able to engage in more traditional forms of cardio exercise. Through faster-paced sequences and certain breathing techniques, practitioners can experience an increase in heart rate, contributing to cardiovascular health and aiding in calorie burn.

- **Dynamic Movements:** By incorporating sequences that involve dynamic movements, such as seated sun salutations or modified flow sequences, practitioners can elevate their heart rate, promoting cardiovascular endurance and contributing to calorie expenditure.
- **Breathing Exercises:** Pranayama, or yogic breathing exercises, can also play a role in cardiovascular health. Techniques such as Kapalabhati (skull shining breath) are invigorating and can increase heart rate, offering a form of cardio workout that is suitable for those who may be seated or require the support of a chair.

Mindful Eating and Stress Reduction

Chair Yoga extends beyond physical activity, incorporating elements of mindfulness and stress reduction that can indirectly support weight loss efforts. The practice encourages a mindful approach to eating and a reduction in stress, both of which are crucial for making healthier food choices and managing calorie intake.

- **Encouragement of Mindful Eating:** The mindfulness cultivated through Chair Yoga practice can extend to eating habits, encouraging practitioners to eat slowly, savor their food, and recognize signals of fullness. This mindful approach can prevent overeating and promote satisfaction with smaller portions, contributing to a caloric deficit necessary for weight loss.
- **Stress Reduction:** High stress levels are linked to weight gain, particularly due to the production of the hormone cortisol, which can increase appetite and fat storage in the

abdominal area. Regular Chair Yoga practice helps reduce stress and lower cortisol levels, mitigating stress-related eating and supporting weight management efforts.

Practical Implementation for Weight Loss

Incorporating Chair Yoga into a weight loss routine involves consistency and a holistic approach to health. Practitioners are encouraged to engage in regular sessions, aiming for at least 20-30 minutes per day, and to combine their practice with a balanced, nutritious diet. As Chair Yoga promotes increased body awareness and mindfulness, individuals may find themselves more attuned to their dietary needs and more motivated to make healthful food choices.

Conclusion

Chair Yoga proves to be an effective tool for weight loss, offering a multifaceted approach that stimulates metabolism, provides cardiovascular conditioning, and supports mindful eating practices. Its accessibility and adaptability make it an appealing option for a wide range of individuals, including those who may be new to exercise or have limitations that make traditional workouts challenging. By integrating Chair Yoga into a comprehensive lifestyle approach that includes healthy eating and regular activity, individuals can achieve sustainable weight loss and improve their overall well-being.

Benefits of Chair Yoga

Chair Yoga emerges as a beacon of inclusivity and adaptability within the vast expanse of yoga practices, particularly beneficial for seniors and individuals with mobility issues. This gentle form of yoga, which adapts traditional poses for execution with the aid of a chair, provides a myriad of health benefits that transcend mere physical well-being to include mental and emotional health. This comprehensive exploration delves into the numerous advantages Chair Yoga offers, emphasizing its impact on daily activities for seniors, its inherent safety, and its holistic contributions to a healthier lifestyle.

Enhancing Daily Activities for Seniors

Improved Flexibility and Mobility: One of the most immediate benefits seniors may notice from practicing Chair Yoga is an enhancement in flexibility and mobility. The range of motion in joints such as the shoulders, hips, and knees can significantly improve, making daily tasks—such as reaching for items on a high shelf or bending to tie shoelaces—more manageable and less strenuous.

Increased Strength and Balance: Regular Chair Yoga practice strengthens the body's core muscles as well as those in the arms and legs. This increase in strength directly impacts balance, a critical concern for seniors, as it reduces the risk of falls. Enhanced strength and balance support independence in daily activities, from carrying groceries to navigating stairs with confidence.

Pain Management: Chair Yoga offers therapeutic exercises that can alleviate pain and discomfort associated with conditions such as arthritis, osteoporosis, and chronic back pain. The gentle stretching and strengthening movements improve circulation and reduce stiffness, making it easier for seniors to engage in their daily routines without being hampered by chronic pain.

Safety and Accessibility of Chair Yoga for Seniors

Low Risk of Injury: The seated or supported nature of Chair Yoga poses minimizes the risk of falls and injuries, making it a safe exercise option for seniors. The chair provides stability and support, allowing practitioners to focus on their form and breath without the fear of losing balance.

Adaptability to Individual Needs: Chair Yoga can be easily modified to accommodate individual health conditions and mobility levels. Whether a senior is recovering from surgery or managing a chronic health issue, poses can be adapted to ensure safety and comfort, making Chair Yoga a highly inclusive practice.

Promotion of Joint Health: The gentle movements encouraged in Chair Yoga are beneficial for joint health, lubricating joints and increasing synovial fluid, which helps in easing movements and reducing discomfort from conditions like arthritis.

Holistic Health Benefits of Chair Yoga

Cardiovascular Health: Regular participation in Chair Yoga can contribute to cardiovascular health by reducing blood pressure and improving circulation. The combination of physical postures and deep breathing exercises enhances heart efficiency, offering a protective benefit against heart disease.

Stress Reduction and Mental Clarity: Chair Yoga incorporates mindfulness and breathing techniques that promote relaxation and stress reduction. These practices can lower cortisol levels, mitigate the effects of stress on the body, and enhance mental clarity, improving overall quality of life.

Enhanced Respiratory Function: The emphasis on breathing techniques in Chair Yoga improves lung capacity and respiratory function. For seniors, especially those with respiratory conditions, this can lead to better oxygenation of the body, increased energy levels, and improved immune function.

Social Engagement and Community: Joining Chair Yoga classes provides an opportunity for social interaction, reducing feelings of loneliness and isolation among seniors. The shared experience of yoga fosters a sense of community and belonging, which is crucial for mental and emotional health.

Integrating Chair Yoga into Daily Life

Consistency is Key: To reap the full benefits of Chair Yoga, consistency in practice is crucial. Seniors incorporating Chair Yoga into their routine, even if for a few minutes daily, can experience significant improvements in their physical and mental well-being.

Seeking Professional Guidance: For those new to Chair Yoga, starting with professional guidance can ensure the practice is both safe and effective. Yoga instructors trained in Chair Yoga can provide personalized modifications and support to address individual needs and goals.

Incorporating Mindfulness: Beyond the physical poses, integrating the mindfulness and meditation aspects of Chair Yoga into daily life can enhance emotional resilience and provide tools for managing stress and anxiety.

Conclusion

Chair Yoga stands out as a profoundly beneficial practice for seniors, addressing a wide spectrum of physical, mental, and emotional health concerns. Its adaptability ensures that individuals at various levels of mobility and health can safely participate and reap its myriad benefits. By improving flexibility, strength, balance, and mental clarity, Chair Yoga enhances the quality of daily life for seniors, fostering independence and a greater sense of well-being. Moreover, its emphasis on safety, combined with the holistic health benefits it offers, makes Chair Yoga an essential component of a healthy aging strategy, empowering seniors to lead active, fulfilling lives.

CHAPTER 1.
STRETCHING AND BREATHING EXERCISES

Embarking on a journey into the realms of stretching and breathing exercises opens the door to a world where balance, wellness, and tranquility converge. This introduction is designed to guide you through the preparatory steps necessary to engage in these exercises effectively, anticipate the sensations and benefits you may experience, and understand the profound impact they can have on your overall well-being.

Preparing for Stretching and Breathing Exercises

Creating a Conducive Environment: To begin, choose a quiet, comfortable space where distractions are minimized. This could be a corner of your living room, a dedicated exercise room, or even a peaceful spot outdoors. The environment should invite calmness, allowing you to focus inwardly during your practice.

Choosing the Right Time: While stretching and breathing exercises can be performed at any time of day, consider scheduling your practice at a time when you're least likely to be interrupted. Many find early morning or evening to be ideal, as these times naturally lend themselves to reflection and relaxation.

Wearing Comfortable Clothing: Opt for loose, breathable clothing that doesn't restrict movement. Comfort in attire will enable you to perform stretches more effectively and enjoy a deeper, more unrestricted flow of breath.

Gathering Necessary Props: While not always necessary, certain props can enhance your practice. A yoga mat provides cushioning and grip for floor exercises, while a blanket or bolster can support various poses. A sturdy chair can also be invaluable for seated stretches or as a prop for balance.

Setting Intentions: Before beginning, take a moment to set an intention for your practice. This could be anything from seeking relaxation, improving flexibility, or simply dedicating time to self-care. Setting an intention helps to focus your mind and infuse your practice with purpose.

During the Exercise: Sensations and Mindfulness

Tuning Into Your Breath: As you move through the exercises, maintain a focus on your breathing. Each inhale and exhale should be deliberate, helping to guide your movements and deepen your stretches. The breath acts as a bridge between the body and mind, anchoring you in the present moment.

Listening to Your Body: Pay close attention to the sensations in your body, approaching your limits with kindness and respect. Stretching should induce a feeling of gentle tension rather than pain. If discomfort arises, ease back and adjust your posture or the intensity of the stretch.

Embracing Stillness and Movement: While some exercises invite stillness, others involve gentle, flowing movements. Embrace both aspects, allowing yourself to enjoy the stillness and engage with the dynamic stretches that bring energy and vitality.

After the Exercise: Reflection and Benefits

Reflecting on Your Experience: After completing your stretching and breathing exercises, take a few moments to reflect on how you feel. You may notice a sense of calm, a release of tension, or a renewed sense of energy. This reflection helps to connect the physical practice with its emotional and psychological benefits.

Physical Benefits: Regular practice can lead to increased flexibility, improved posture, and enhanced physical balance. These exercises also promote better circulation and can help in alleviating muscle stiffness and pain, contributing to a more comfortable and agile body.

Mental and Emotional Benefits: Stretching and breathing exercises are profoundly calming, offering a respite from the stresses of daily life. They can improve mental clarity, reduce symptoms of anxiety and depression, and promote a sense of groundedness. The focus on breath helps to regulate the nervous system, encouraging a state of relaxation and well-being.

Incorporating Practice into Daily Life: To fully reap the benefits, consider making these exercises a consistent part of your daily routine. Even a few minutes each day can make a significant difference in your physical health and mental state.

Stretching and breathing exercises are much more than mere physical activities; they are a holistic practice that nurtures the body, soothes the mind, and enriches the spirit. As you embark on this journey, remember that the goal is not perfection but progress and self-discovery. With regular practice, you will not only witness improvements in your flexibility and respiratory function but also experience a profound enhancement in your overall quality of life. Let this be a journey of exploration, where each breath and stretch brings you closer to your inner self, fostering a sense of peace and well-being that permeates every aspect of your being.

A comprehensive guide for "5 Stretching and Breathing Exercises of Chair Yoga" with tutorials and benefits for each exercise, tailored to seniors or those with mobility issues, requires attention to detail and a deep understanding of the practice's impact on physical and mental well-being. Here's an in-depth exploration of these exercises, highlighting the steps involved and the myriad benefits they offer.

1. Seated Mountain Pose with Deep Breathing

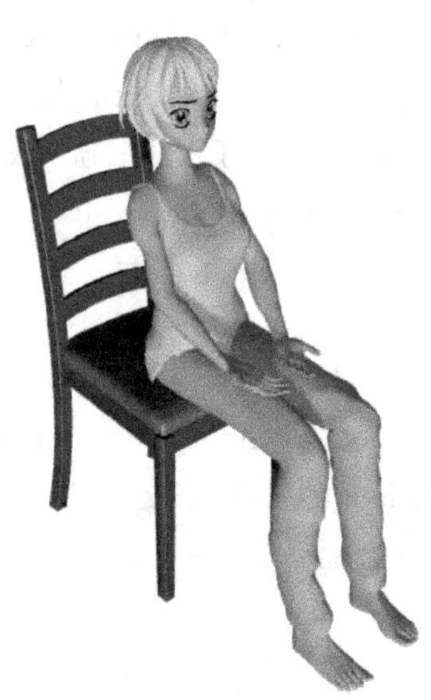 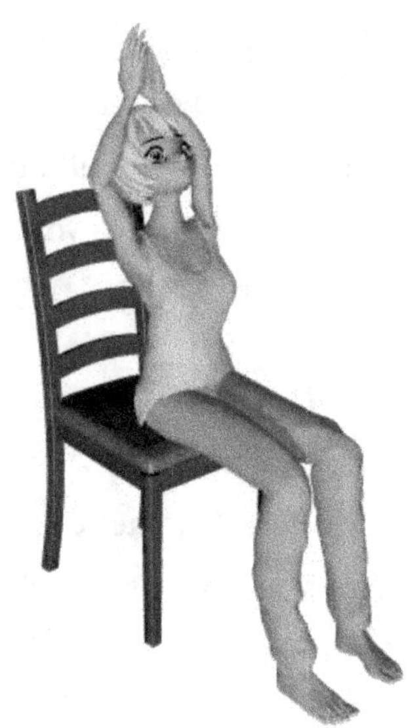

Tutorial:

- Begin by sitting at the edge of a sturdy chair, feet flat on the floor, spine long, and hands resting on your knees or thighs.
- Inhale deeply, elongating your spine as if a string were pulling you up from the crown of your head. Exhale slowly, maintaining the length in your spine.
- With each inhalation, raise your arms overhead, palms facing each other. With each exhalation, slowly lower your arms back to your sides.
- Repeat this movement for 3-5 minutes, focusing on deep, controlled breaths that fill your chest and abdomen.

Benefits:

- Enhances lung capacity and improves respiratory function.
- Promotes a sense of grounding and stability.
- Improves posture and spinal alignment.
- Reduces stress and calms the mind through focused breathing.

2. Seated Cat-Cow Stretch

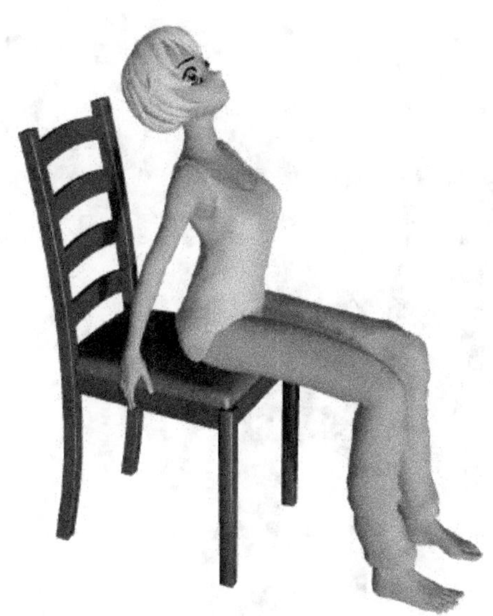 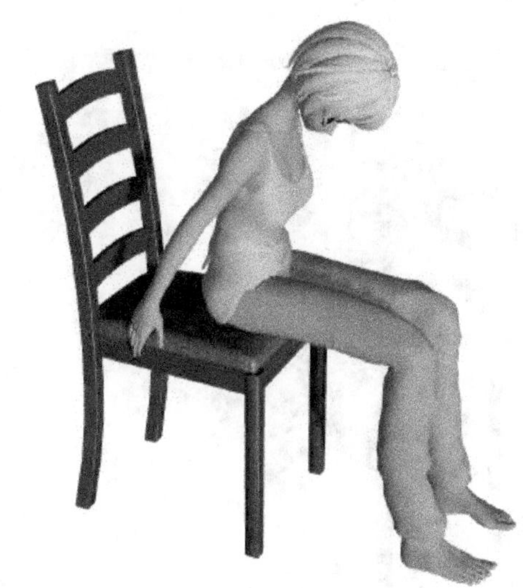

Tutorial:

- Sit at the edge of your chair, feet flat on the ground, hands on your knees.
- Inhale, arch your back, and look up towards the ceiling, pushing your chest forward for the Cow position.
- Exhale, round your spine, tucking your chin to your chest, pulling your belly in for the Cat position.
- Flow between these two positions for 3-5 minutes, allowing your breath to guide the movement.

Benefits:

- Increases flexibility in the spine and neck.
- Stimulates the digestive tract and spinal fluid.
- Enhances coordination of breath and movement, promoting mental clarity.

3. Chair Pigeon Pose

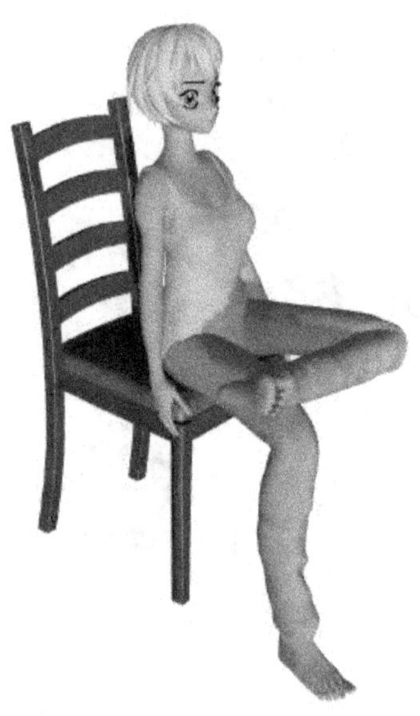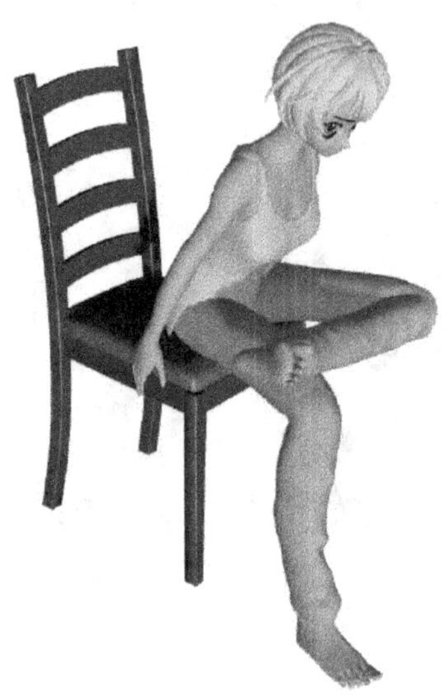

Tutorial:

- Sitting firmly on the chair, place your right ankle over your left knee, keeping the right knee open to the side.
- Maintain an upright spine; gently lean forward from the hips, increasing the stretch as you breathe deeply.
- Hold this position for 1-2 minutes, then switch legs and repeat.
- Focus on breathing deeply throughout, relaxing into the stretch with each exhale.

Benefits:

- Opens the hips and stretches the glutes and piriformis muscle.
- Reduces lower back pain and tension.
- Improves mobility and flexibility in the lower body.
- Encourages deep breathing, aiding in stress reduction.

4. Seated Twist

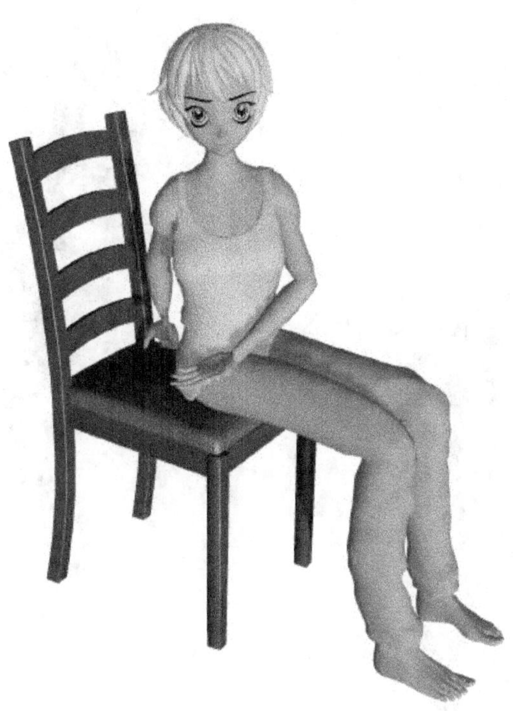

Tutorial:

- Sit upright with your feet flat on the floor. Place your left hand on your right knee and your right hand behind you on the seat of the chair.
- Inhale to lengthen your spine, and as you exhale, gently twist to the right, looking over your right shoulder.
- Hold this position for 30 seconds to 1 minute, breathing deeply, then slowly return to center and repeat on the opposite side.

Benefits:

- Stimulates digestion and helps detoxify the organs.
- Improves spinal mobility and flexibility.
- Reduces spinal compression and can alleviate back pain.
- Encourages a deeper sense of relaxation through focused breathing.

5. Seated Forward Bend

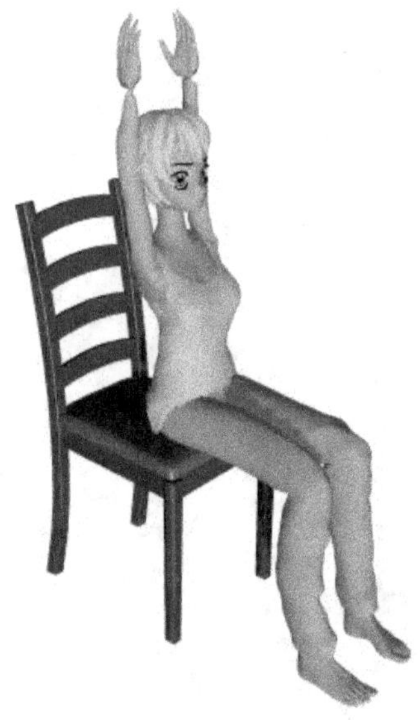 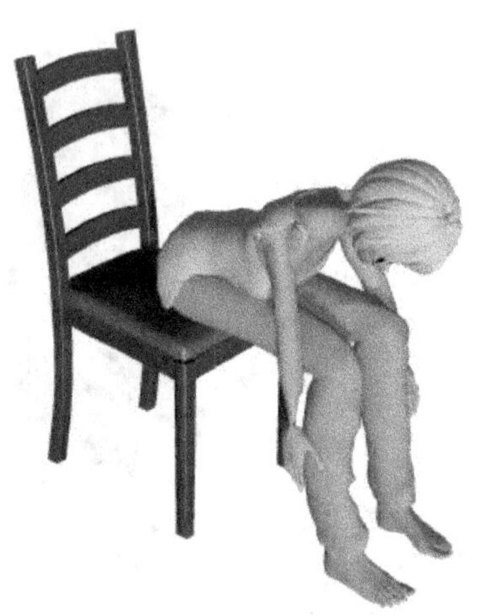

Tutorial:

- Begin seated, inhale and extend your arms overhead. As you exhale, hinge at your hips and bend forward, lowering your hands towards your feet.
- Allow your hands to rest wherever they reach comfortably; on your shins, ankles, or the floor.
- Keep your spine long and neck relaxed, breathing deeply in this position for 1-2 minutes before slowly rising back to a seated posture.

Benefits:

- Stretches the spine, shoulders, and hamstrings.
- Calms the brain, relieving stress and mild depression.
- Stimulates the liver, kidneys, ovaries, and uterus.
- Improves digestion and soothes headache and anxiety symptoms.

These exercises, integral to Chair Yoga, are designed to be accessible, safe, and highly beneficial for seniors. They contribute to improved flexibility, strength, and mental well-being, making daily activities more manageable and enhancing overall quality of life. Regular practice can lead to significant improvements in health, mobility, and mood, underscoring Chair Yoga's value as a comprehensive, gentle fitness regimen.

CHAPTER 2.
CHAIR YOGA EXERCISES

Chair Yoga represents a transformative approach to wellness, adapting the ancient practice of yoga to be accessible and beneficial for everyone, regardless of age, mobility, or fitness level. This form of yoga utilizes a chair as a tool or prop to modify traditional yoga poses, making the practice inclusive and adaptable. The following introduction aims to guide you through the initial steps to embark on Chair Yoga exercises, describe the potential feelings during and after the practice, and elucidate the myriad benefits it brings.

Preparing for Chair Yoga Exercises

Creating Your Space: Choose a quiet, comfortable spot where you can place your chair on a stable, flat surface. This could be in your living room, bedroom, or any area that offers enough space to move freely. The ambiance of your chosen space can significantly impact your practice, so consider soft lighting or natural light and perhaps an open window for fresh air.

Selecting the Right Chair: The ideal chair for Chair Yoga is sturdy, without wheels, and without arms. This ensures your safety during exercises and allows for a range of movements without restriction. The chair should support your weight fully and provide a stable base for both seated and standing poses.

Wearing Appropriate Clothing: Opt for comfortable, flexible clothing that doesn't restrict your movements. The right attire will allow you to perform various stretches and poses without discomfort, enhancing your overall experience.

Setting Aside Time: Dedicate a specific time of day for your Chair Yoga practice, considering when you feel most energized or in need of relaxation. Consistency in practice is key to experiencing the full benefits, so try to incorporate it into your daily routine, even if for only a few minutes at a time.

Gathering Additional Props: While not always necessary, having a yoga mat, strap, or block can be helpful, especially for certain poses or to add support and comfort. These can be used in conjunction with the chair to modify poses or assist in achieving deeper stretches.

During Chair Yoga: Experiences and Sensations

Engaging Fully with the Practice: As you move through the Chair Yoga poses, focus on your breath and the sensations in your body. Chair Yoga encourages mindfulness and present-moment awareness, which can deepen your practice and enhance its benefits.

Listening to Your Body: Pay attention to your body's signals. Chair Yoga is designed to be gentle and accessible, but it's important to avoid pushing yourself too hard. If you feel pain or discomfort, gently ease out of the pose or adjust your alignment. The goal is to find a balance between effort and ease.

Finding Joy in Movement: Chair Yoga can be surprisingly dynamic and enjoyable. Allow yourself to find pleasure in the movements and the unique way your body can stretch and strengthen with the support of the chair. This positive engagement can significantly enhance your emotional well-being.

After Chair Yoga: Reflections and Benefits

Physical and Mental Refreshment: Many practitioners report feeling physically refreshed and mentally clearer after a Chair Yoga session. The combination of stretching, strengthening, and breathing exercises can leave you feeling more energized and yet deeply relaxed.

Increased Mobility and Flexibility: Regular Chair Yoga practice can lead to noticeable improvements in flexibility and mobility. This can have a profound impact on daily life, making activities that were once challenging or uncomfortable much easier and more enjoyable.

Stress Reduction and Emotional Balance: One of the most cherished benefits of Chair Yoga is its ability to reduce stress and promote emotional equilibrium. The mindful breathing and meditative aspects of the practice encourage a state of calm and can help manage anxiety and depression.

Improved Strength and Balance: Chair Yoga not only enhances flexibility but also builds strength, particularly in the core, arms, and legs. This increased strength contributes to better balance and stability, reducing the risk of falls and injuries.

Enhanced Overall Well-being: Beyond the physical benefits, Chair Yoga promotes an overall sense of well-being. The practice fosters a deeper connection between mind, body, and spirit, contributing to a heightened sense of peace, contentment, and vitality.

Chair Yoga is a powerful practice that demystifies yoga, making it accessible and enjoyable for all. It stands as a testament to the adaptability and inclusiveness of yoga, offering a pathway to improved physical health, mental clarity, and emotional resilience. As you integrate Chair Yoga into your life, you may discover not just the physical benefits but also a deeper sense of connection to yourself and the world around you. Whether you're seeking to enhance your mobility, reduce stress, or simply find a new way to engage with yoga, Chair Yoga offers a safe, effective, and fulfilling way to nurture your well-being.

An extensive guide for "5 Chair Yoga Exercises" distinct from stretching and breathing routines previously outlined involves crafting detailed instructions and highlighting the unique benefits each pose offers. This guide aims to provide seniors and individuals with limited mobility a diverse set of exercises that enhance physical health and overall well-being.

1. Chair Warrior II

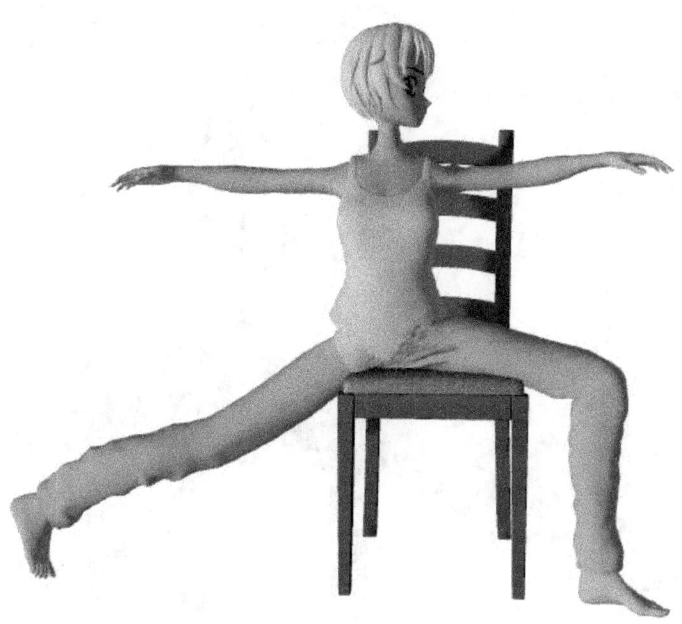

Tutorial:

- Start by sitting sideways on the chair, with your left side facing the back of the chair. Extend your left leg back, keeping your foot flat on the floor, and bend your right knee at a 90-degree angle, foot planted firmly on the ground.
- Open your arms wide, reaching them out to the sides, parallel to the floor, gaze over your right hand.
- Keep your torso upright and your spine straight, breathing deeply. Hold this position for 30 seconds to 1 minute, then switch sides and repeat.

Benefits:

- Strengthens the legs, ankles, and feet while stretching the groins, chest, and lungs.
- Enhances stamina and concentration.
- Stimulates abdominal organs, aiding in digestion.
- Promotes a sense of balance and grounding.

2. Chair Extended Side Angle

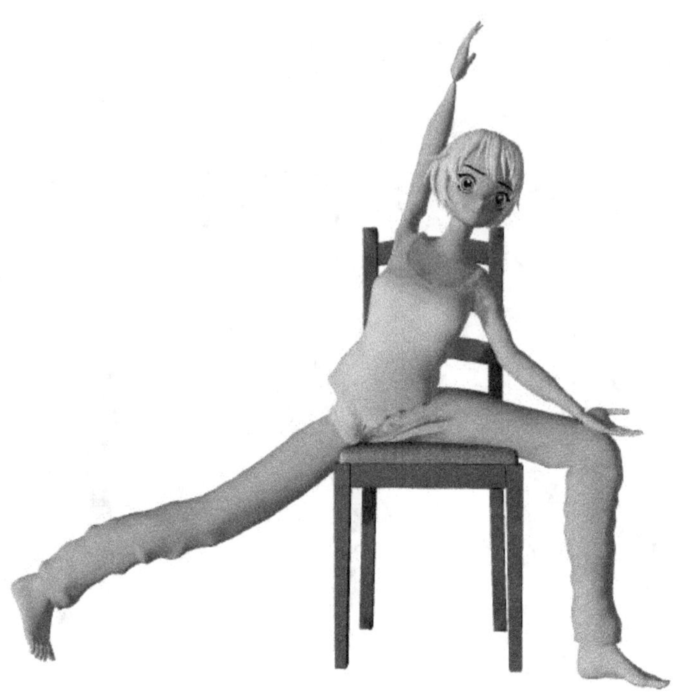

Tutorial:

- Remain seated sideways as with Warrior II, with your right leg bent and left leg extended back.
- Place your right forearm on your right thigh and extend your left arm over your left ear, creating a straight line from your left foot through the left fingertips.
- Turn your head to look up under your left arm, keeping your chest open and shoulders stacked. Hold for 30 seconds to 1 minute, then switch sides and repeat.

Benefits:

- Stretches the sides of the body, improving flexibility in the spine.
- Opens the chest and shoulders, aiding in respiratory functions.
- Stimulates abdominal organs, improving digestion.
- Enhances concentration and balance, fostering a mental and physical equilibrium.

3. Chair Eagle Arms

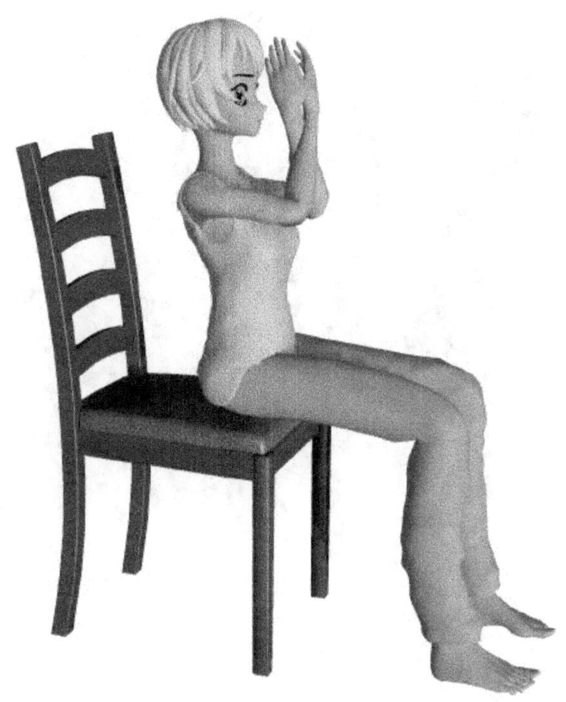

Tutorial:

- Sit upright in your chair, feet flat on the floor, arms extended at shoulder height.
- Cross your right arm over your left, bending both elbows. Twist your arms so your palms come together, or as close as possible.
- Lift your elbows while dropping your shoulders away from your ears. Hold this position for 30 seconds to 1 minute, focusing on deep breaths, then switch arms and repeat.

Benefits:

- Relieves tension in the shoulders and upper back.
- Improves concentration and balance.
- Enhances joint mobility in the wrists, elbows, and shoulders.
- Stimulates the lymphatic system, aiding in the removal of toxins.

4. Chair Child's Pose

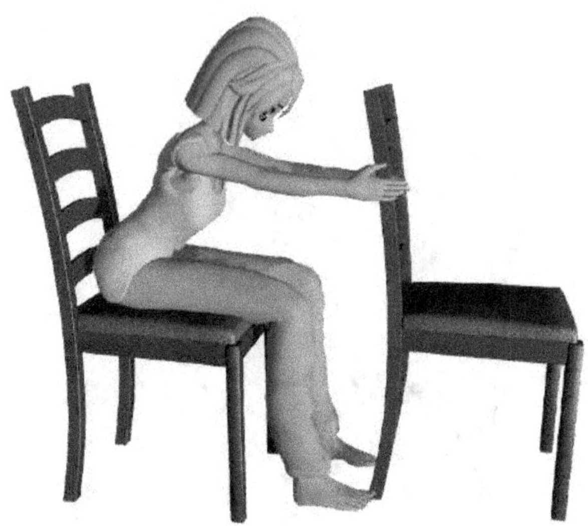

Tutorial:

- Place two chairs facing each other. Sit on one chair. Place a folded towel on the other's seat and ensure it is within reach.
- Now, take a deep breath and elongate your spine.
- As you breathe out, bend your upper torso forward until your arms comfortably rest on the other chair's seat. While doing this, ensure your arms are outstretched and not bent at the elbows.
- Hold this pose for up to a minute while breathing slowly and deeply.
- After this, slowly get back to the initial position.

Benefits:

- Enhances spinal flexibility and relieves back tension.
- Stimulates digestive organs, aiding in digestion and detoxification.
- Reduces stress and calms the nervous system.
- Improves posture and alignment of the spine.

5. Chair Savasana

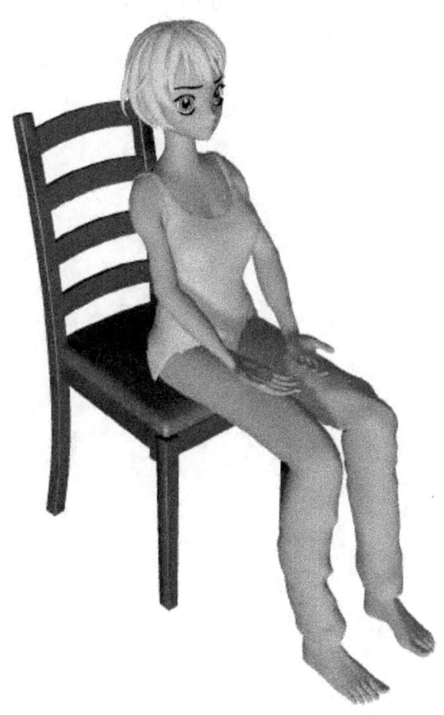

Tutorial:

- Sit comfortably in your chair, feet flat on the floor, hands on your lap or by your sides, palms facing up.
- Close your eyes and take deep, slow breaths. Relax every part of your body, from your head down to your toes, releasing tension with each exhale.
- Stay in this relaxed state for 5-10 minutes, allowing your mind to become calm and clear.

Benefits:

- Deeply relaxes the body and reduces stress.
- Lowers blood pressure and slows the heart rate, promoting heart health.
- Enhances mental clarity and focus.
- Rejuvenates the body and mind, preparing you for the rest of your day or a good night's sleep.

These five Chair Yoga exercises provide a comprehensive approach to improving physical health, flexibility, and mental well-being. Regular practice can lead to noticeable improvements in strength, balance, and overall quality of life, making them a valuable addition to any senior's daily routine.

CHAPTER 3.
FOCUS ON ARMS AND SHOULDERS

Arm and shoulder exercises are essential components of a comprehensive fitness routine, designed to strengthen, tone, and enhance the mobility of the upper body. These exercises target various muscle groups, including the biceps, triceps, deltoids, and rotator cuff muscles, contributing to improved functionality and aesthetics of the arms and shoulders. This introduction will guide you through the preparatory steps for engaging in arm and shoulder exercises, the sensations you might experience during and after the workout, and the myriad benefits that accompany a dedicated upper body regimen.

Preparing for Arm and Shoulder Exercises

Creating a Suitable Environment: Choose a space that is conducive to focused exercise, whether it's a corner of your living room, a home gym, or even outdoors. Ensure there's enough room to move your arms freely in all directions without obstruction.

Selecting Appropriate Equipment: Depending on the specific exercises you plan to incorporate, you may need equipment such as dumbbells, resistance bands, a stability ball, or even just your body weight. Choose tools that match your current fitness level; starting with lighter weights or resistance bands can help prevent injury.

Wearing the Right Attire: Comfortable, non-restrictive clothing is crucial, as you'll be moving your arms and shoulders extensively. Opt for fabrics that wick away moisture to keep you cool and dry during your workout.

Warm-Up: A proper warm-up is essential to prepare your muscles and joints for the workout ahead. Spend 5-10 minutes on light aerobic activity, such as walking or jogging in place, followed by dynamic stretches that specifically target the arms and shoulders.

Setting Realistic Goals: Before beginning, set clear, achievable goals for your arm and shoulder workouts. Whether you're aiming to increase muscle strength, improve endurance, or enhance muscle tone, having specific objectives can help keep you motivated and focused.

During the Exercise: Sensations and Engagement

Mind-Muscle Connection: Pay close attention to the muscles you're engaging during each exercise. Focusing on the sensation of muscle contraction and movement can enhance the effectiveness of the workout and prevent injury.

Breathing: Proper breathing is crucial. Exhale during the exertion phase of the exercise and inhale during the easier phase. This not only helps with performance but also ensures you're supplying your muscles with ample oxygen.

Pacing Yourself: It's important to perform each exercise with control, rather than rushing through the movements. A slower pace allows for better muscle engagement and reduces the risk of swinging or using momentum, which can lead to injuries.

After the Exercise: Reflection and Recovery

Cool Down and Stretch: After completing your arm and shoulder exercises, take time to cool down with light aerobic activity to gradually lower your heart rate. Follow this with static stretches focusing on the arms and shoulders to enhance flexibility and reduce muscle soreness.

Hydration and Nutrition: Replenish your body by drinking plenty of water and consuming a balanced meal or snack. Protein is particularly important for muscle repair and recovery, so consider including a source of high-quality protein in your post-workout nutrition.

Listening to Your Body: It's normal to feel some muscle fatigue and soreness after a workout, especially in the beginning. However, sharp pain or discomfort is not normal and may indicate overexertion or injury. Pay attention to your body's signals and allow adequate rest and recovery between workout sessions.

Benefits of Arm and Shoulder Exercises

Increased Strength and Endurance: Regular training leads to stronger, more resilient arm and shoulder muscles, enhancing performance in various physical activities and daily tasks.

Improved Posture and Stability: Strong shoulders and upper back muscles contribute to better posture, which can reduce the risk of back pain and other musculoskeletal issues.

Enhanced Aesthetics: Toned arms and shoulders can significantly improve your body's appearance, boosting confidence and self-esteem.

Functional Benefits: Strong arms and shoulders are crucial for lifting, carrying, and performing a wide range of motions necessary for daily life, making these exercises not just about aesthetics but also about improving quality of life.

Injury Prevention: Strengthening the muscles and tendons around the shoulders can help protect against injuries, particularly those related to overuse and repetitive motion.

Arm and shoulder exercises are pivotal for building strength, enhancing mobility, and improving the overall function of the upper body. By properly preparing for your workout, engaging mindfully during each exercise, and focusing on recovery afterward, you can maximize the benefits of your regimen. Whether your goals are related to fitness, functionality, or aesthetics, incorporating regular arm and shoulder exercises into your routine can lead to significant improvements in your health, well-being, and quality of life.

A detailed guide for "5 Chair Yoga Exercises for Arms and Shoulders" tailored for seniors or those with mobility challenges ensures a focus on improving strength, flexibility, and reducing discomfort in these areas. Each exercise is designed to be accessible, safe, and beneficial, providing clear tutorials and outlining the unique advantages of incorporating these movements into a regular practice.

1. Seated Shoulder Circles

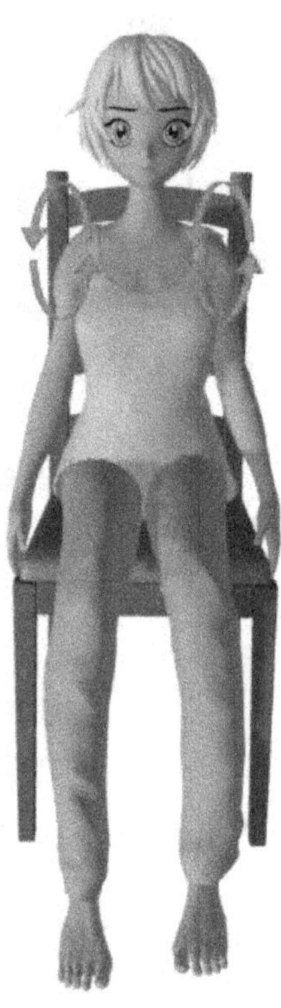

Tutorial:

- Sit comfortably in your chair, feet flat on the floor, spine straight.
- Relax your arms by your sides and slowly begin to roll your shoulders in a forward circular motion.
- After 30 seconds, reverse the direction, rolling your shoulders backward.
- Perform this movement for 3-5 minutes, focusing on smooth, controlled motions.

Benefits:

- Increases mobility and flexibility in the shoulders.
- Reduces tension and stiffness in the upper back and neck.
- Improves circulation and lymphatic flow around the shoulder area.
- Encourages relaxation and stress relief through gentle movement.

2. Chair Arm Raises

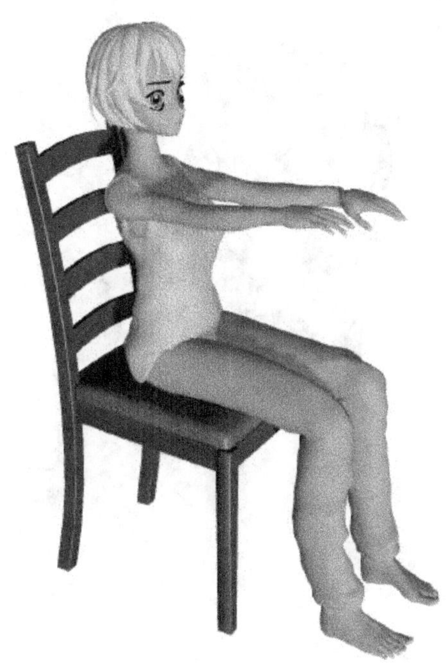

Tutorial:

- Sit upright with your feet planted firmly on the ground.
- Extend your arms straight in front of you at shoulder height, palms facing down.
- Inhale and slowly raise your arms upward, keeping them straight, until your hands are pointing towards the ceiling.
- Exhale and gently lower your arms back to the starting position.
- Repeat this movement for 3-5 minutes, focusing on a fluid motion and deep breathing.

Benefits:

- Strengthens the shoulders, arms, and upper back.
- Enhances joint flexibility and range of motion in the shoulders.
- Promotes better posture by engaging and strengthening the upper body.
- Boosts concentration and mental focus through coordinated movement and breathing.

3. Modified Goddess Pose

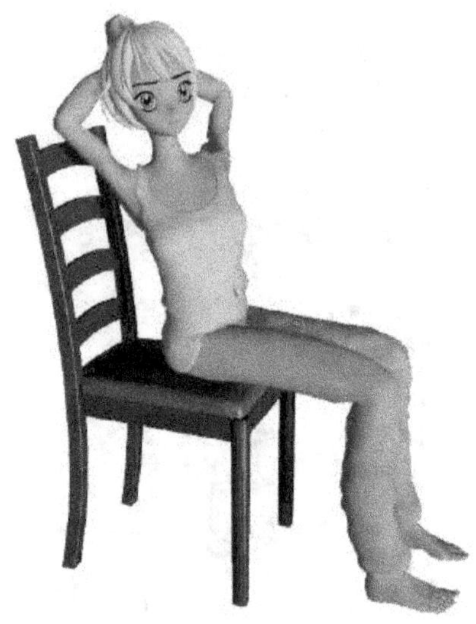

Tutorial:

- Begin by comfortably sitting in a chair with your back straight and shoulders relaxed. Ensure your feet are firmly planted on the floor with your hands resting on your thighs.

- Breathe in slowly and deeply while moving your legs apart until you notice a slight stretch. While doing this, ensure your knees and ankles are perfectly aligned with your toes pointing outward. Bend your hands at the elbow and move them behind your head. Lace your fingers together for added support.

- As you breathe out, gently move your upper torso to the left so the left elbow points to the floor.

- Breathe in and gently move back to the sitting position. After this, repeat it on the other side.

Benefits:

- Stretches and opens the shoulder joints, improving flexibility.
- Relieves tension in the shoulders, neck, and upper back.
- Enhances arm and shoulder strength through isometric tension.
- Promotes focus and mental clarity by requiring concentration on balance and posture.

4. Seated Scapular Retraction

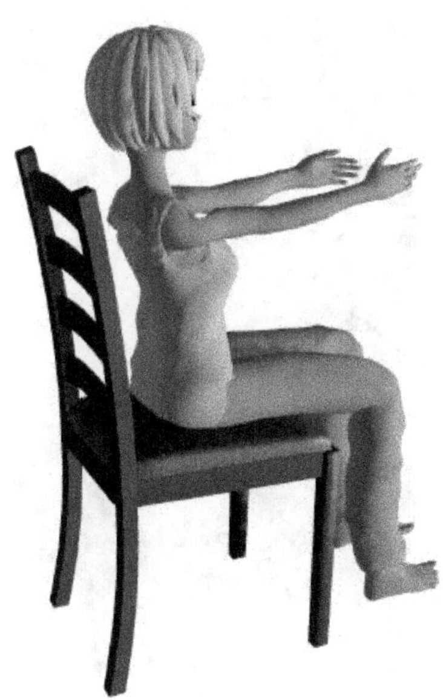

Tutorial:

- Sit at the edge of your chair with your feet flat on the ground and your spine tall.
- Extend your arms in front of you at shoulder height, palms facing each other.
- Draw your shoulder blades together as you pull your elbows back, aiming to squeeze them towards each other behind you.
- Hold this squeeze for 5 seconds, then slowly extend your arms back to the starting position.
- Repeat for 3-5 minutes, concentrating on the engagement of your shoulder blades and upper back.

Benefits:

- Strengthens the muscles between the shoulder blades, improving posture.
- Reduces risk of shoulder injuries by enhancing scapular stability and mobility.
- Alleviates tension and pain in the upper back and shoulders.
- Encourages deep breathing, which can reduce stress and improve oxygen flow to muscles.

5. Seated Arm Twists

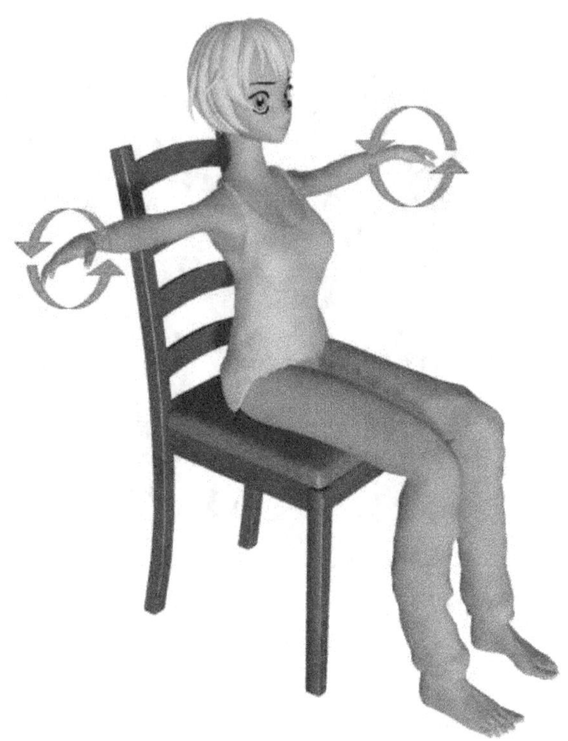

Tutorial:

- Sit upright in your chair, feet firmly planted on the floor.
- Extend your arms out to the sides at shoulder height, palms facing down.
- Keeping your arms at shoulder height, rotate your arms so that your palms face up, then rotate them back down.
- Continue this movement, twisting your arms from the shoulders, for 3-5 minutes.

Benefits:

- Improves rotational mobility and flexibility in the shoulders.
- Strengthens the arm muscles, including the biceps, triceps, and forearm muscles.
- Enhances coordination and proprioception (body awareness).
- Stimulates blood flow to the upper body, nourishing the shoulder joints and muscles.

These five exercises specifically target the arms and shoulders, making them ideal for seniors seeking to maintain or improve upper body strength, flexibility, and reduce discomfort. Regular practice can lead to significant improvements in mobility, ease daily activities, and enhance overall well-being. Each exercise combines physical movement with focused breathing, emphasizing the holistic benefits of Chair Yoga for physical health and mental clarity.

CHAPTER 4.
FOCUS ON LEGS AND CALVES

Legs and calves exercises are foundational components of a balanced fitness regimen, targeting some of the largest muscle groups in the body. These exercises are crucial not only for athletes but for anyone looking to enhance their overall physical health, improve functional strength, and boost their metabolism. This introduction will guide you through the preparation required for a legs and calves workout, the sensations you might experience during and after the session, and the extensive benefits that stem from focusing on these lower body muscles.

Preparing for Legs and Calves Exercises

Creating an Optimal Environment: Choose a space where you have enough room to move freely, ensuring safety and effectiveness in your workout. Whether you're at home, in a gym, or outdoors, the area should allow for a full range of motion for all exercises.

Selecting the Right Equipment: Depending on your workout plan, you might need various equipment pieces, such as dumbbells, kettlebells, a resistance band, or a barbell. However, many leg and calf exercises can also be performed using just your body weight, making them accessible regardless of your setting.

Appropriate Attire: Wear comfortable, flexible clothing that won't restrict your movements, along with supportive footwear that offers stability and grip. Proper shoes are particularly important for leg workouts to prevent slips and provide a solid foundation for lifting.

Warm-Up: A dynamic warm-up is essential to prepare your muscles and joints for the intensity of a legs and calves workout. Incorporate movements such as leg swings, ankle circles, and light jogging to increase blood flow and reduce the risk of injury.

Hydration and Nutrition: Ensure you're well-hydrated before starting your workout and keep water nearby to sip during the session. Additionally, consider your pre- and post-workout nutrition to fuel your body adequately for recovery and muscle growth.

During the Exercise: Engagement and Sensations

Mindful Movement: Focus on each exercise's form and technique rather than speed or the amount of weight lifted. Proper form ensures maximum efficiency and safety, helping to prevent injury.

Pacing Yourself: Legs and calves exercises can be particularly taxing due to the large muscle groups involved. Pay attention to your body's signals, taking breaks when needed and adjusting the intensity of your workout accordingly.

Breathing: Maintain a consistent breathing pattern, inhaling during less strenuous parts of the movement and exhaling during the exertion phase. Proper breathing supports performance and oxygen delivery to your muscles.

After the Exercise: Recovery and Reflection

Cool Down: Gradually reduce the intensity of your activity with a cool-down period, followed by stretching the muscles you've worked. Stretching can help alleviate post-workout soreness and improve flexibility.

Post-Workout Sensations: It's normal to feel muscle fatigue and soreness in the days following a rigorous leg and calf workout, known as delayed onset muscle soreness (DOMS). This is a sign your muscles are adapting and strengthening.

Nutrition and Hydration: Rehydrate and refuel your body with a meal or snack rich in proteins and carbohydrates to aid muscle repair and replenish energy stores. Proper nutrition significantly impacts your recovery and the gains from your workout.

Benefits of Legs and Calves Exercises

Enhanced Muscle Strength and Tone: Regular legs and calves workouts build strength in the lower body, contributing to leaner, more toned muscles. This not only improves your appearance but also enhances your physical capabilities in daily activities and sports.

Boosted Metabolism: Working large muscle groups increases calorie burn both during and after exercise, contributing to fat loss and improved body composition over time.

Improved Balance and Stability: Strong legs and calves are essential for balance and stability, reducing the risk of falls and injuries, especially as we age.

Increased Functional Strength: The strength gained from these exercises translates into easier performance of everyday activities, such as climbing stairs, lifting heavy objects, and walking longer distances.

Better Posture: Strong lower body muscles support a proper posture, which can alleviate lower back pain and improve overall spinal health.

Enhanced Athletic Performance: For athletes, strong legs and calves are crucial for nearly every sport, offering improved power, speed, and endurance.

Legs and calves exercises form the cornerstone of a comprehensive fitness program, offering wide-ranging benefits from enhanced physical appearance to improved functional strength and health. By adequately preparing for your workout, focusing on form and technique during the session, and prioritizing recovery afterward, you can maximize the effectiveness of your legs and calves training. Whether your goals are aesthetic, functional, or health-related, incorporating regular lower body workouts into your fitness regimen can lead to significant improvements in your overall well-being and quality of life.

A detailed guide for "5 Chair Yoga Exercises for Legs and Calves" involves creating specific exercises aimed at strengthening, stretching, and improving the flexibility and circulation in the lower limbs. These exercises are particularly beneficial for seniors or individuals with limited mobility, focusing on safe, accessible movements that can be performed with a chair. Each exercise description provides step-by-step instructions followed by a comprehensive list of benefits, ensuring a thorough understanding of their impact on health and well-being.

1. Seated Leg Lifts

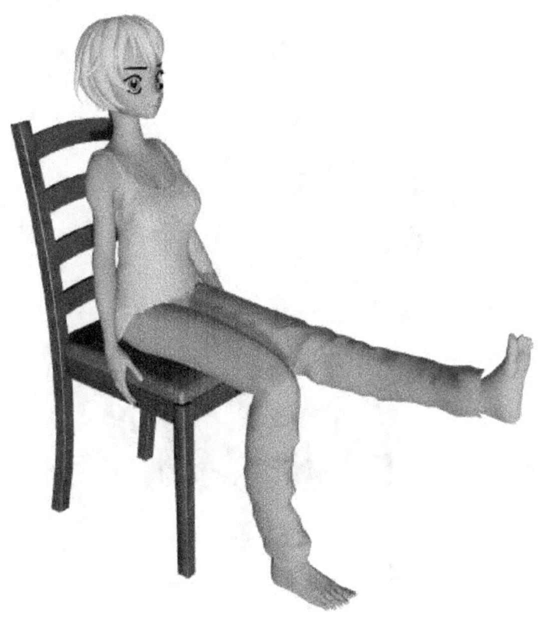

Tutorial:

- Sit upright in your chair, feet flat on the floor, and hands resting on the sides of the chair for support.
- Engage your core and slowly lift your right leg straight out in front of you, keeping the knee straight but not locked. Lift as high as comfortable, aiming for parallel to the floor.
- Hold the lift for a few seconds, then slowly lower your leg back to the starting position.
- Repeat 10-15 times for each leg, focusing on controlled movements.

Benefits:

- Strengthens the quadriceps and hip flexors, improving leg strength and stability.
- Enhances joint flexibility and mobility in the knees and hips.
- Promotes better circulation in the lower extremities, reducing swelling and the risk of blood clots.
- Encourages core engagement and balance, contributing to improved posture and spinal health.

2. Seated Calf Raises

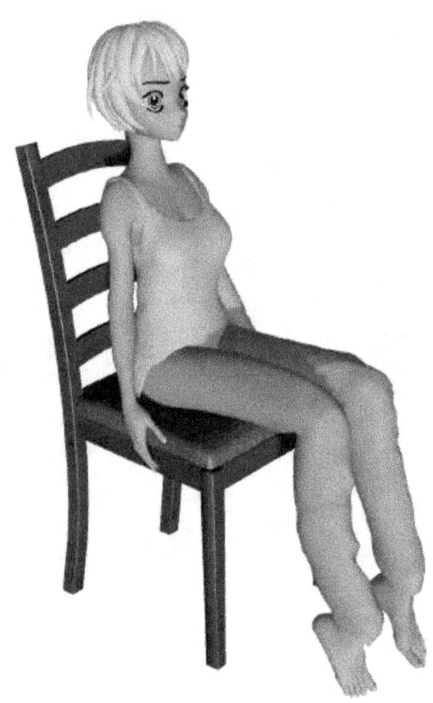

Tutorial:

- Sit towards the edge of the chair with your feet flat on the ground and your hands on your thighs or holding onto the sides of the chair for balance.
- Press down into the balls of your feet and lift your heels as high as possible, squeezing the calf muscles at the top of the movement.
- Hold the raised position for a moment, then slowly lower your heels back to the floor.
- Perform 15-20 repetitions, maintaining a smooth and controlled motion throughout.

Benefits:

- Strengthens the calf muscles, enhancing lower leg strength and stability.
- Improves ankle mobility and flexibility, reducing the risk of falls.
- Aids in pumping blood back up to the heart, improving venous circulation.
- Can help relieve symptoms of restless leg syndrome and reduce leg cramps.

3. Seated Ankle Circles

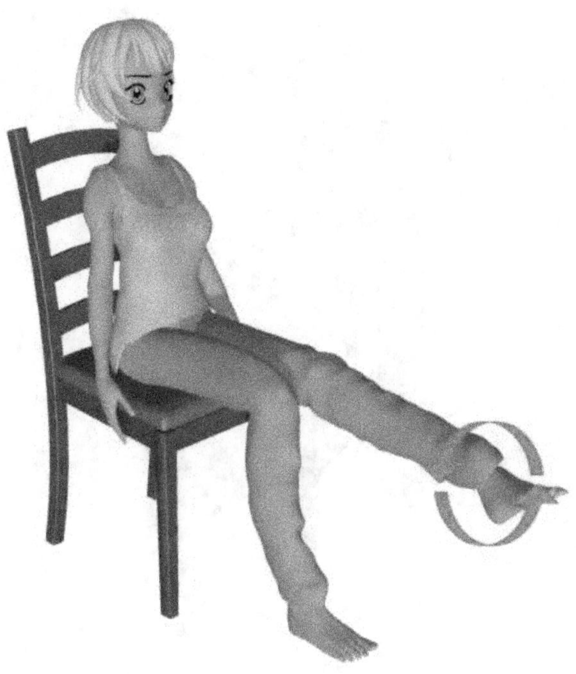

Tutorial:

- Remain seated with your feet flat on the ground. Extend one leg out straight in front of you, holding it off the floor.
- Point your toes and begin to rotate your foot in a circular motion, making as large a circle as possible.
- After 10-15 seconds, reverse the direction of the rotation.
- Repeat with the other foot, ensuring both sides receive equal attention.

Benefits:

- Enhances flexibility and range of motion in the ankle joint.
- Reduces stiffness and discomfort in the ankles, especially for those who experience arthritis or swelling.
- Promotes better circulation in the feet and lower legs.
- Encourages focus and mental clarity through the coordination of movement and breath.

4. Chair Marching

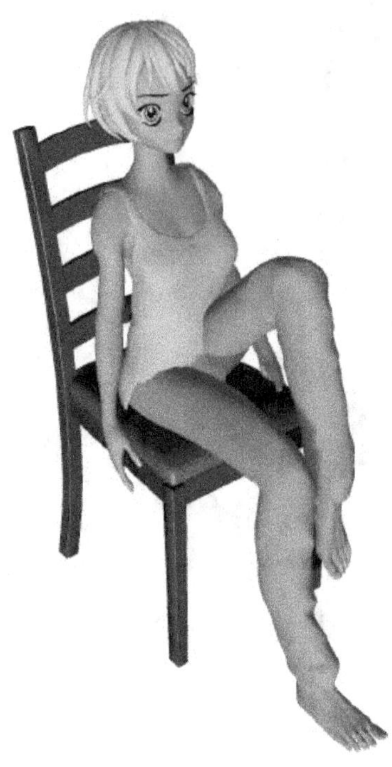

Tutorial:

- Sit up straight in your chair with your feet flat on the floor and your hands resting on your thighs or holding the sides of the chair.
- Lift your right knee towards your chest as high as comfortably possible, then place it back down. Repeat with your left knee, alternating as if marching in place.
- Continue this alternating knee lift for 1-2 minutes, maintaining an upright posture throughout.

Benefits:

- Strengthens the hip flexors and core muscles, improving stability and balance.
- Increases heart rate slightly, providing a mild cardiovascular workout.
- Enhances coordination and stimulates neural connections between the brain and legs.
- Can alleviate lower back pain by strengthening the supporting muscles around the spine.

5. Seated Knee Extensions

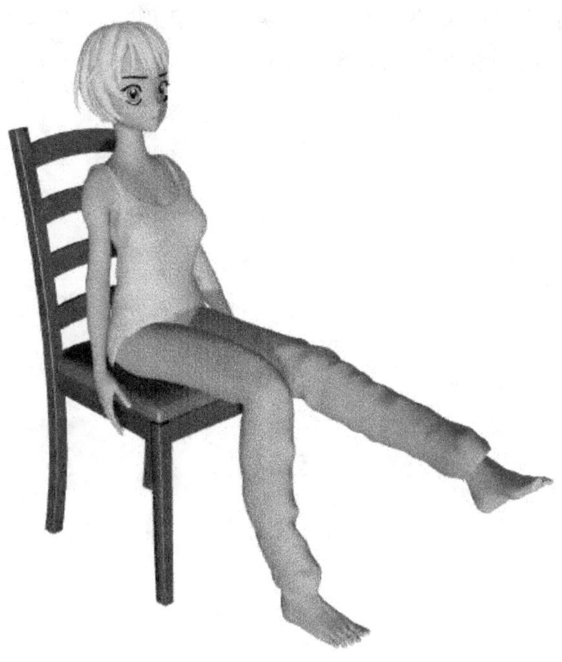

Tutorial:

- Sit in a chair with your feet flat on the floor, hands on the sides of the chair or on your thighs.
- Extend one leg at a time, straightening the knee as much as possible, and flex your foot to point your toes towards you.
- Hold the extension for a few seconds, then slowly lower your leg back to the starting position.
- Repeat 10-15 times for each leg, focusing on a smooth, controlled motion.

Benefits:

- Strengthens the quadriceps, which are crucial for knee stability and strength.
- Promotes flexibility in the knee joints, aiding in the prevention of stiffness and injury.
- Encourages better circulation in the legs, supporting overall cardiovascular health.
- Engages the core and improves posture through mindful, controlled movements.

47

These five exercises offer a comprehensive approach to improving leg and calf strength, flexibility, and circulation, tailored to be safe and accessible for seniors and individuals with mobility challenges. Regular practice of these chair yoga exercises can lead to significant improvements in mobility, stability, and overall quality of life, making daily activities easier and reducing the risk of falls and injuries.

CHAPTER 5.
FOCUS ON HIPS AND GLUTES

Hips and glutes exercises stand as pivotal components of a comprehensive fitness regime, targeting crucial muscles that are instrumental in executing a wide array of movements. From walking and climbing stairs to maintaining balance and posture, the strength and flexibility of your hips and glutes affect almost every motion your body makes throughout the day. This introduction is designed to prepare you for engaging in exercises focused on these essential areas, outline the sensations and benefits you might experience, and highlight the significance of these exercises for enhancing daily activities and overall well-being.

Preparing for Hips and Glutes Exercises

Creating a Conducive Space: Select an area where you have enough room to move freely. Your chosen space should be free of obstacles, providing a safe environment for a variety of movements. Whether you're indoors with a mat or in a grassy outdoor area, ensure the surface is stable and non-slip.

Choosing Your Equipment: While many hips and glutes exercises require no equipment, incorporating items like resistance bands, dumbbells, or a stability ball can intensify your workout. Select tools that align with your fitness level and the specific exercises you plan to perform.

Dressing Appropriately: Wear clothing that allows for extensive movement without restriction, particularly around the hips and thighs. Supportive footwear is crucial, even if you're exercising at home, to provide a solid foundation for your movements and protect your feet during standing exercises.

Warming Up: A dynamic warm-up focusing on the lower body is essential to prepare your muscles and joints for the workout. Include exercises that increase your heart rate and enhance mobility in your hips and glutes, such as leg swings, squats, and lunges.

Setting Realistic Goals: Approach your hips and glutes workout with clear, achievable goals. Whether you're aiming to improve strength, enhance muscle tone, or increase flexibility, having specific objectives can motivate you and guide your exercise selection.

During the Exercise: Engagement and Sensations

Focusing on Form: Proper technique is crucial to ensure the effectiveness of each exercise and to prevent injury. Pay close attention to your alignment and the quality of your movements, making adjustments as necessary to maintain correct form.

Monitoring Intensity: Listen to your body and adjust the intensity of your workout according to your current fitness level and how you're feeling on any given day. It's better to perform exercises correctly at a lower intensity than to risk injury by pushing too hard.

Breathing: Maintain a steady, rhythmic breathing pattern throughout your workout. Proper breathing not only aids in performance but also helps you stay focused and centered during your exercise routine.

After the Exercise: Recovery and Reflection

Cooling Down: Gradually decrease the intensity of your activity, transitioning into a cool-down period that includes static stretching, particularly focusing on the hips and glutes. This helps to reduce muscle soreness and improve flexibility.

Hydration and Nutrition: Drink plenty of water to rehydrate after your workout and consume a balanced meal or snack. Nutrients like protein and carbohydrates are vital for muscle repair and recovery, aiding in the development of stronger, more resilient muscles.

Evaluating Sensations: It's normal to experience muscle fatigue and mild soreness after a vigorous hips and glutes workout. This discomfort should be manageable and should diminish over the next few days as your muscles recover and adapt.

Benefits of Hips and Glutes Exercises for Daily Activities

Enhanced Movement Efficiency: Strong hips and glutes contribute to better movement patterns in daily activities, reducing the effort required for walking, climbing stairs, and bending.

Improved Posture and Balance: These exercises strengthen the muscles that support your spine, promoting better posture and balance. This can lead to a reduction in back pain and a lower risk of falls.

Increased Joint Protection: Strengthening the muscles around your hips and glutes helps to stabilize your joints, providing protection against injuries and wear and tear.

Boosted Athletic Performance: For athletes, strong hips and glutes are fundamental for power generation, speed, and agility, enhancing performance in a wide range of sports.

Aesthetic Benefits: In addition to functional benefits, hips and glutes exercises can also improve the shape and tone of your lower body, boosting confidence and body image.

Hips and glutes exercises offer profound benefits that extend far beyond the gym, impacting nearly every aspect of your daily life and physical health. By preparing adequately for your workout, focusing on form and technique during your exercises, and prioritizing recovery afterward, you can unlock the full potential of your lower body's strength and mobility. Whether your goals are functional, aesthetic, or health-related, incorporating regular hips and glutes exercises into your fitness routine can lead to significant improvements in your quality of life, enabling you to move through your days with greater ease, confidence, and resilience.

An in-depth guide for "5 Chair Yoga Exercises for Hips and Glutes" involves detailing exercises specifically designed to enhance the strength, flexibility, and stability of the hip and gluteal regions. These exercises are essential for improving mobility, balance, and overall well-being, particularly for seniors or individuals with limited mobility. Through carefully outlined tutorials and a thorough explanation of benefits, this guide aims to provide valuable insights into each exercise's impact on health and daily functioning.

1. Seated Hip Openers

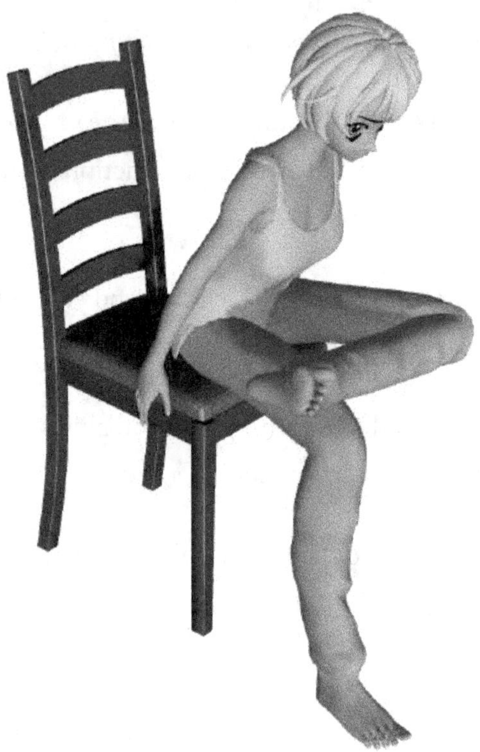

Tutorial: Begin by sitting at the edge of your chair, feet flat on the ground, hip-width apart. Carefully lift your right foot and place it on your left knee, forming a figure-four shape. Keep your back straight, and gently lean forward from your hips, increasing the stretch in your right hip. Hold this position for 30 seconds to 1 minute, feeling a gentle stretch in your hip and glute area. Slowly return to the starting position and repeat on the other side.

Benefits:

- Increases flexibility and range of motion in the hips.
- Reduces tension and tightness in the hip flexors and glutes.
- Aids in the prevention of lower back pain by alleviating pressure on the lumbar spine.
- Enhances circulation in the lower body, promoting healing and reducing swelling.

2. Seated Leg Cross

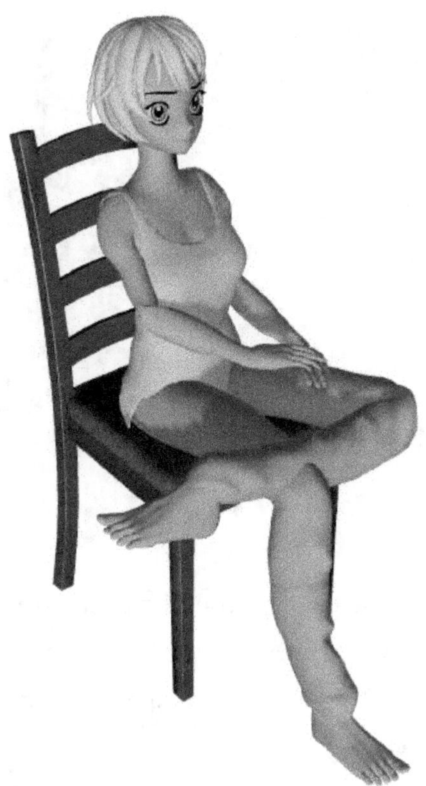

Tutorial: Sit upright with your feet flat on the floor. Cross your right leg over your left, fully resting your right ankle on your left knee. Maintain a straight spine as you gently press down on your right knee, intensifying the stretch. For a deeper stretch, lean slightly forward from the hips, keeping your back straight. Hold this position for 30 seconds to 1 minute, then switch legs and repeat.

Benefits:

- Targets the outer hips and glutes, improving flexibility and relieving tightness.
- Promotes synovial fluid production in the hip joints, enhancing mobility.
- Can alleviate symptoms of sciatica and reduce hip discomfort.
- Encourages mindfulness and relaxation through focused stretching and breathing.

3. Chair Pigeon Pose

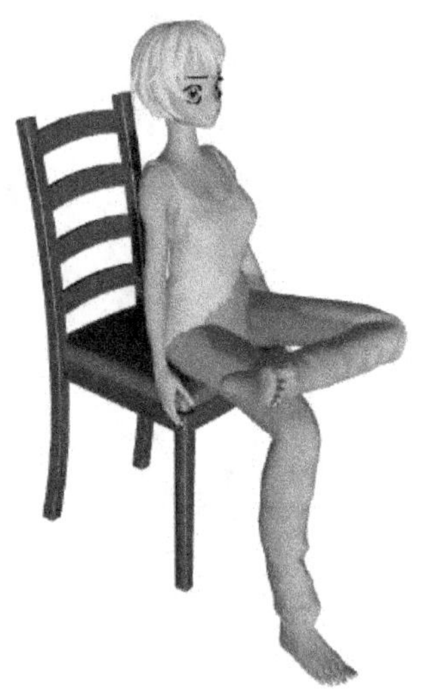 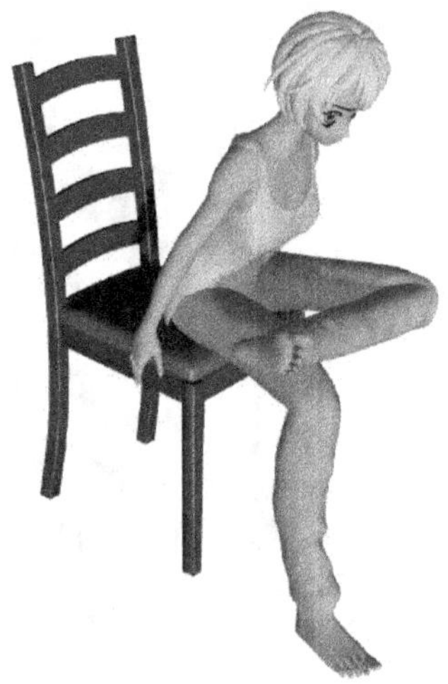

Tutorial: While seated, place your right ankle on your left knee, creating a figure-four shape. Ensure your right knee is pointing sideways. Gently lean forward, keeping your back straight and engaging your core. This position should create a stretch in your right hip and glute. Hold for 30 seconds to 1 minute, then carefully switch to the other side.

Benefits:

- Deeply stretches the hip rotators and glutes, aiding in flexibility and range of motion.
- Helps alleviate lower back and sciatic pain by releasing tension in the hip area.
- Enhances pelvic stability, contributing to better posture and balance.
- Stimulates the abdominal organs, potentially aiding in digestion.

4. Seated Marching Hip Lifts

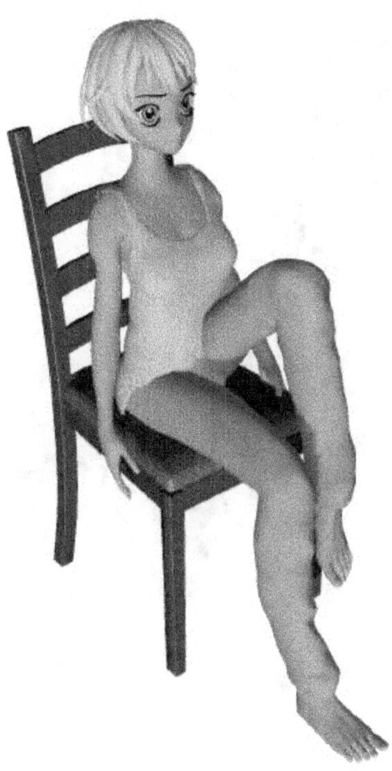

Tutorial: Sit at the edge of your chair with your feet flat on the ground. Place your hands on the sides of the chair for support. Lift your right knee towards your chest as much as possible, then place it back down. Repeat with your left knee, alternating in a marching motion. For added challenge, press into your planted foot to lift your hips slightly off the chair as you march.

Benefits:

- Strengthens the hip flexors, improving mobility and stability.
- Activates the core and glutes, enhancing posture and lower back support.
- Increases circulation to the lower extremities, promoting overall leg health.
- Improves coordination and balance, reducing the risk of falls.

5. Seated Side Leg Raises

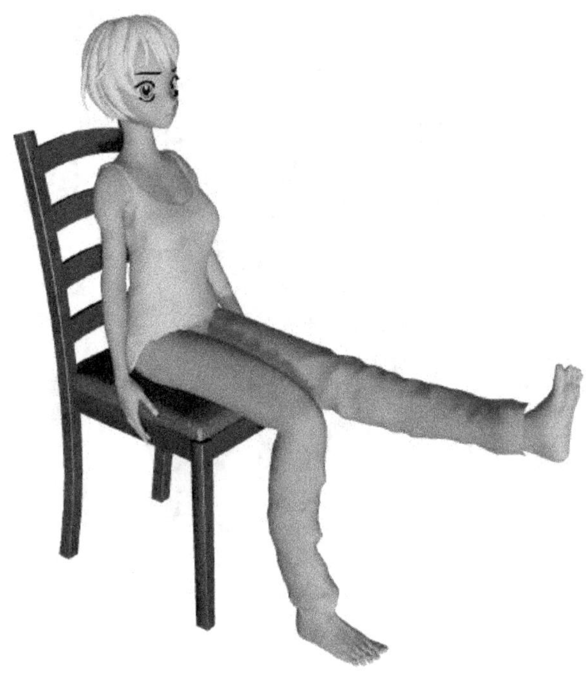

Tutorial: Sit on the chair with your feet flat and hands resting on your lap or holding the sides of the chair. Shift your weight slightly to the left side, and straighten your right leg out to the side as much as possible. Lift your right leg to the side, keeping it straight, then lower it back down. Perform 10-15 repetitions before switching to the left leg.

Benefits:

- Targets and strengthens the abductor muscles and glutes, supporting hip stability.
- Enhances lateral mobility and flexibility, important for daily activities like walking and climbing stairs.
- Reduces the risk of hip and knee injuries by strengthening surrounding muscles.
- Promotes balance and body awareness, crucial for maintaining independence in daily activities.

These five chair yoga exercises for the hips and glutes are designed to be both accessible and effective, offering a safe way to improve strength, flexibility, and balance. Regular practice can significantly impact overall mobility and quality of life, making everyday movements easier and reducing the risk of injury. This comprehensive approach ensures that individuals can enjoy the benefits of yoga, regardless of their mobility level, in a safe and supportive manner.

CHAPTER 6.
CARDIO FOCUS

Cardiovascular exercise, often simply referred to as cardio, is a cornerstone of physical fitness, especially for seniors. It encompasses any activity that increases heart rate and blood circulation throughout the body, enhancing the overall function of the heart, lungs, and circulatory system. For seniors, engaging in regular cardio activities can significantly improve health, mobility, and quality of life. This introduction aims to guide you through the initial steps to engage in cardio exercises safely, manage your heart rate during exercise, understand the sensations you might experience, and uncover the manifold benefits, particularly for daily activities.

Preparing for Cardio Exercise

Choosing the Right Environment: Begin by selecting a suitable and safe environment for your cardio workout. Whether it's a brisk walk in the park, a session on a stationary bike at home, or a water aerobics class at the local pool, the setting should be conducive to sustained physical activity and free from hazards.

Wearing Appropriate Attire: Comfort is key when it comes to exercise gear. Opt for breathable, moisture-wicking fabrics to keep you cool and shoes with good support and non-slip soles to minimize the risk of falls.

Hydration is Crucial: Start well-hydrated and keep water within reach during your workout. Staying hydrated helps prevent fatigue and overheating, ensuring you can complete your session safely.

Warm-Up: A proper warm-up is essential to prepare your body for the increased activity level. Spend 5-10 minutes doing gentle movements such as walking at a slow pace, arm circles, or leg swings. This helps gradually raise your heart rate and loosen up your muscles.

Consultation with a Healthcare Provider: Particularly for those with pre-existing health conditions, it's wise to consult with a healthcare provider before starting any new exercise regimen. They can offer personalized advice based on your health status and fitness level.

During the Exercise: Managing Heart Rate and Engagement

Monitoring Your Heart Rate: Keeping an eye on your heart rate ensures you're working within a safe range. Use a heart rate monitor or periodically check your pulse manually. The target heart rate zone for seniors during moderate-intensity activities is typically 50-70% of your maximum heart rate.

What to Do If Your Heart Rate Goes Up: If you notice your heart rate is higher than recommended, slow down or take a break. It's crucial to listen to your body and not push beyond what feels comfortable. Rest until your heart rate returns to a more manageable level before continuing at a slower pace.

Staying Mindful: Pay attention to how your body feels throughout the exercise. It's normal to experience an increase in breathing rate, but you should still be able to speak. If you find yourself out of breath, slow down to reduce intensity.

After the Exercise: Recovery and Reflection

Cool Down: Gradually reduce the intensity of your activity to bring your heart rate down gently. Follow up with stretches to help prevent stiffness and soreness, focusing on flexibility and relaxation.

Hydrate and Refuel: Drink water to rehydrate after your session, and consider a snack or meal that includes carbohydrates and protein to help your body recover.

Notice How You Feel: Many seniors report feeling energized and more alert after cardio exercise. You may also notice improvements in sleep quality and mood due to the endorphins released during physical activity.

Benefits for Daily Activities

Improved Cardiovascular Health: Regular cardio exercise strengthens the heart and lungs, reducing the risk of heart disease, high blood pressure, and stroke. A strong cardiovascular system ensures that daily tasks are less taxing.

Enhanced Mobility and Independence: Cardio activities help maintain and improve mobility, balance, and muscle strength, crucial factors in preserving independence in senior years.

Increased Energy Levels: Regular physical activity boosts stamina, making it easier to engage in daily activities without excessive fatigue.

Better Mental Health: Cardio exercise has been shown to reduce symptoms of anxiety and depression, enhance cognitive function, and improve overall emotional well-being.

Social Opportunities: Many cardio exercises for seniors, such as walking groups or water aerobics classes, provide valuable opportunities for social interaction, reducing feelings of loneliness and isolation.

Cardio exercise offers a wealth of benefits for seniors, touching on aspects of physical health, mental and emotional well-being, and social life. By preparing properly, paying attention to your body's signals during exercise, and focusing on recovery afterward, you can safely enjoy the advantages of increased activity. Whether you're looking to improve your health, maintain your independence, or simply enjoy the outdoors, incorporating regular cardio into your routine can be a game-changer for your overall quality of life.

Designing "5 Cardio-Focused Chair Yoga Exercises" involves creating exercises that increase heart rate and enhance cardiovascular health, all while being accessible and safe for individuals who prefer or require seated workouts. These exercises aim to provide a comprehensive cardiovascular workout, improving heart health, enhancing lung capacity, and boosting overall energy levels.

1. Seated Jacks

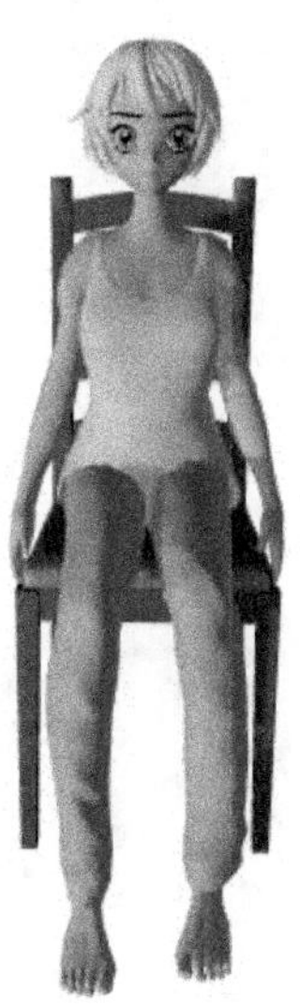 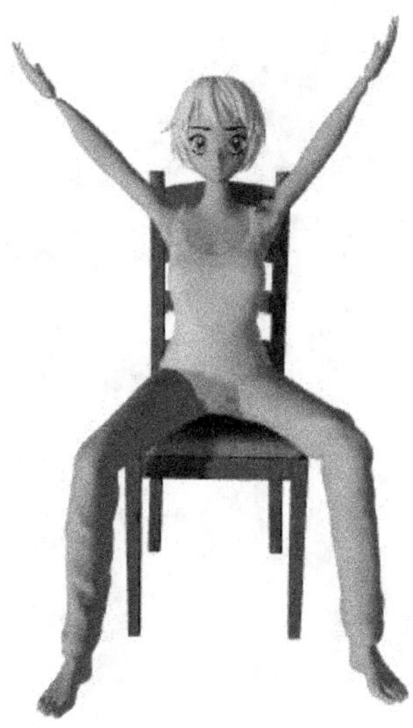

Tutorial:

- Sit on the edge of a sturdy chair with your spine straight, feet flat on the floor, and arms by your side.
- Simultaneously open your legs out to the sides and raise your arms above your head, similar to the motion of a jumping jack but while seated.
- Quickly bring your legs back together and lower your arms to your sides.
- Continue these seated jacks at a brisk pace for 1-2 minutes, focusing on keeping the movements sharp and controlled.

Benefits:

- Increases heart rate, providing a cardiovascular boost similar to standing jumping jacks.
- Improves coordination and stimulates lymphatic flow, aiding in detoxification.
- Enhances muscular endurance in the legs and arms.
- Boosts mood and energy levels through dynamic movement.

2. Chair Marching with Arm Swings

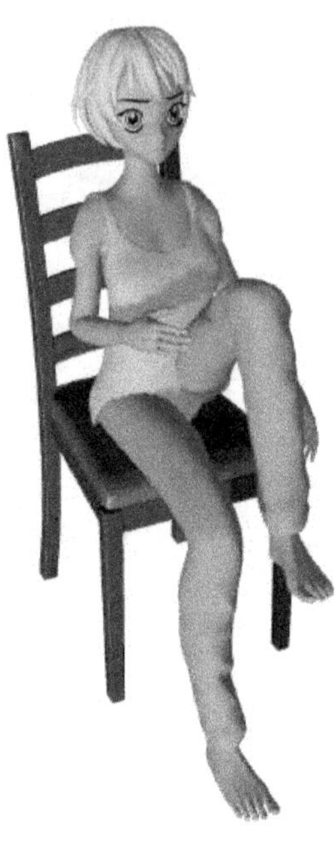

Tutorial:

- Sit up straight with your feet flat on the ground. Begin to march your feet up and down, lifting your knees as high as comfortably possible.
- Add arm swings by alternating your arms forward and backward in opposition to your legs, mimicking the natural motion of walking briskly.
- Continue this exercise for 2-3 minutes, gradually increasing the speed of your marches and arm swings to safely elevate your heart rate.

Benefits:

- Provides a moderate cardiovascular workout, increasing heart rate and improving circulation.
- Strengthens the core and improves balance, reducing the risk of falls.
- Enhances joint mobility in the hips, knees, ankles, and shoulders.
- Energizes the body and clears the mind, making it a great exercise to combat fatigue.

3. Seated Side Steps

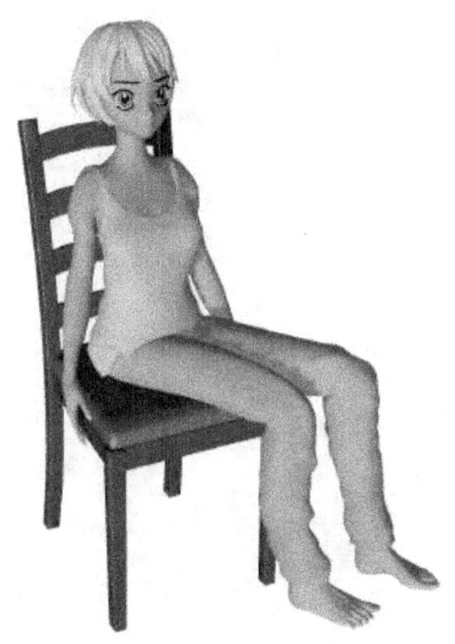 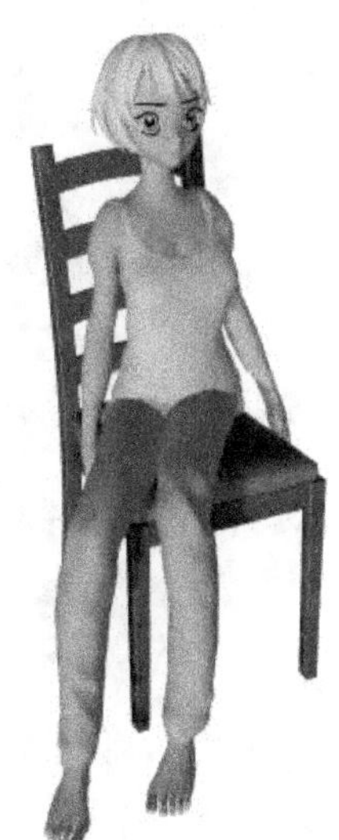

Tutorial:

- Sit at the edge of your chair with your feet together and hands resting on your thighs or holding the edges of the chair for balance.
- Step your right foot out to the side, then step your left foot to meet it, keeping the movement brisk.
- Reverse the movement by stepping your left foot out, then bringing your right foot to meet it.
- Alternate these side steps at a quick pace for 1-2 minutes, engaging your core to maintain posture.

Benefits:

- Activates the side leg muscles, glutes, and core, enhancing lateral movement and stability.
- Improves cardiovascular health by raising the heart rate in a safe, controlled manner.
- Encourages better hip mobility and strengthens the pelvic floor muscles.
- Increases blood flow and reduces stiffness, especially beneficial for those who sit for extended periods.

4. Seated Leg Extensions with Arm Raises

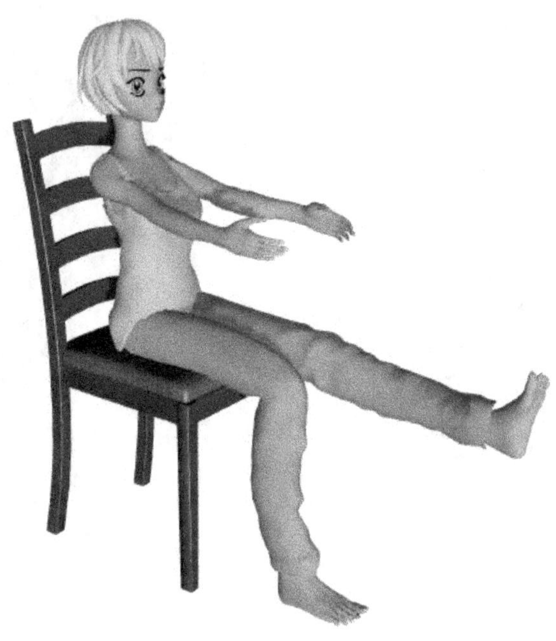

Tutorial:

- Begin seated with feet flat on the floor and arms at your sides.
- Extend one leg at a time in front of you while simultaneously raising both arms in front. Lower your leg and arms, then repeat with the other leg, creating a rhythmic motion.
- Perform this exercise for 2-3 minutes, focusing on extending the leg and arms fully with each repetition to maximize heart rate increase.

Benefits:

- Strengthens the quadriceps, hamstrings, and shoulders, promoting muscular endurance.
- Enhances coordination between leg and arm movements, stimulating neural pathways.
- Provides a cardiovascular challenge that boosts heart health and lung function.
- Increases overall body awareness and posture through balanced, synchronized movements.

5. Chair Tap Dancing

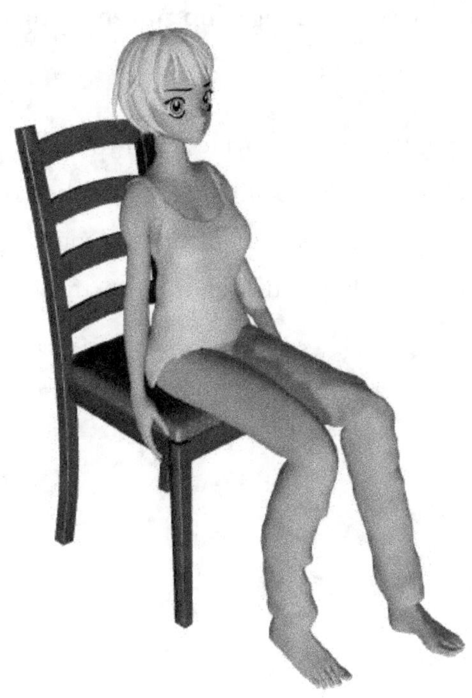

Tutorial:

- Sit on the edge of your chair with feet flat on the floor and hands on your hips or the chair for stability.
- Begin by tapping your feet on the floor rapidly, alternating between left and right, mimicking the footwork of tap dancing.
- Incorporate arm movements by tapping your hands on your thighs or clapping to the rhythm of your feet to add intensity.
- Continue this lively movement for 2-3 minutes, maintaining a brisk pace to keep your heart rate up.

Benefits:

- Enhances cardiovascular endurance and increases heart rate, promoting heart health.
- Improves lower leg strength, agility, and coordination, benefiting daily mobility and balance.

- Stimulates cognitive function through rhythm and coordination of complex foot and hand patterns.
- Elevates mood and energy levels, offering a fun and engaging way to incorporate cardio into your routine.

These five cardio-focused chair yoga exercises provide a well-rounded cardiovascular workout that is both accessible and effective for individuals seeking to improve their heart health, increase their energy levels, and enjoy the benefits of an active lifestyle, all from the comfort of a chair. Regular practice can lead to significant improvements in cardiovascular endurance, muscular strength, and overall well-being.

DIETARY TIPS TO MAXIMIZE WEIGHT LOSS

Understanding the basics of nutrition is essential for anyone looking to manage their weight effectively, particularly for seniors who may be engaging in chair yoga as part of their fitness regimen. This comprehensive understanding not only aids in selecting the right foods to fuel the body but also ensures that dietary choices contribute positively to overall health and wellness goals. This section delves into the pivotal role of macronutrients and micronutrients in the body, along with guiding you on how to calculate and interpret your daily caloric needs for weight loss.

The Role of Macronutrients in Energy Production and Muscle Repair

Macronutrients are the cornerstone of our diet, consisting of carbohydrates, proteins, and fats, each playing a unique and vital role in energy production and muscle repair.

- **Carbohydrates** are the body's primary energy source, broken down into glucose which fuels our muscles and brain. For those engaging in physical activities like chair yoga, carbohydrates ensure there is enough energy to perform exercises effectively. Whole grains, fruits, vegetables, and legumes are excellent sources of complex carbohydrates, providing a steady release of energy.
- **Proteins** are crucial for muscle repair and growth. They are made up of amino acids, some of which are essential and must be obtained through diet. As we age, maintaining muscle mass becomes critical for preserving strength and mobility. High-quality protein sources such as lean meats, fish, dairy, legumes, and nuts help in the repair of tissues damaged during exercise, supporting muscle health and recovery.
- **Fats** are often misunderstood, yet they are essential for absorbing vitamins, providing energy, and supporting cell growth. Healthy fats, such as those found in avocados, nuts, seeds, and fish, contribute to energy production, especially during low to moderate-intensity exercise like chair yoga, and aid in the recovery process by reducing inflammation.

The Importance of Micronutrients for Body Function and Disease Prevention

While macronutrients provide the bulk of dietary energy, micronutrients — vitamins and minerals — are crucial for optimizing health, supporting body functions, and preventing diseases.

- **Vitamins** such as Vitamin D, essential for bone health, and Vitamin C, key for immune function, play significant roles in maintaining health and preventing conditions like osteoporosis and infections. Antioxidant vitamins, such as Vitamins A, C, and E, protect the body from oxidative stress, which can damage cells.
- **Minerals** like calcium and magnesium are vital for bone health, whereas iron is crucial for blood production and oxygen transport. Regular intake of a varied diet rich in fruits, vegetables, lean proteins, and whole grains ensures adequate supply of these essential micronutrients, promoting overall health and aiding in the prevention of chronic diseases such as heart disease, diabetes, and cancer.

Calculating and Interpreting Daily Caloric Needs for Weight Loss

Understanding your daily caloric needs is fundamental to weight management. This calculation considers several factors, including age, gender, weight, height, and physical activity level. The Basal Metabolic Rate (BMR) represents the number of calories your body needs at rest to support vital functions. When combined with calories burned through physical activity, you get your Total Daily Energy Expenditure (TDEE).

To lose weight, you'll need to create a caloric deficit, consuming fewer calories than your body expends. A safe and sustainable deficit is typically around 500 calories per day, which can lead to a gradual weight loss of about 1 pound per week. However, it's important to ensure that the caloric intake does not drop too low, which can lead to muscle loss and a decrease in metabolic rate.

- **Calculating BMR and TDEE:** Various formulas can be used to calculate BMR, such as the Harris-Benedict equation or the Mifflin-St Jeor equation, with the latter being noted for its accuracy. Once the BMR is determined, it can be adjusted based on your physical activity level to find your TDEE. Online calculators or a consultation with a healthcare provider can simplify this process.

- **Interpreting Caloric Needs:** Once you know your TDEE, you can plan your diet to ensure a healthy caloric deficit. Incorporating nutrient-dense foods is key to meeting your body's nutritional needs while staying within your caloric limit. This balance supports weight loss while ensuring your body has the nutrients it needs to function optimally.

In conclusion, understanding the basics of nutrition is not just about weight loss; it's about fostering a lifestyle that promotes vitality and wellness. By appreciating the roles of macronutrients and micronutrients and knowing how to calculate and manage caloric intake, individuals can make informed dietary choices that support their health goals. This knowledge is particularly empowering for seniors practicing chair yoga, offering a foundation for nourishing the body and supporting an active, healthy lifestyle.

Embarking on a weight loss journey requires not just an understanding of nutritional basics but also a strategic approach to meal planning. This ensures that every meal contributes positively towards achieving your weight loss goals while also being nutritious and satisfying. In this context, planning your meals can be a transformative practice, incorporating techniques for portion control, the benefits of meal prepping, and the crafting of balanced meals.

Techniques for Effective Portion Control to Manage Calorie Intake

Portion control is fundamental in managing calorie intake, an essential aspect of weight loss. It involves understanding and serving sizes that align with your nutritional needs without overindulging. Here are strategies to master portion control:

- **Use Smaller Plates:** This visually cues you to take less food, naturally reducing calorie intake without feeling deprived.
- **Read Food Labels:** Becoming acquainted with serving sizes on food labels can help you gauge how much of a particular food aligns with your dietary goals.
- **Measure Servings:** Initially, use measuring cups or a kitchen scale to familiarize yourself with recommended serving sizes. Over time, you'll be able to estimate servings more accurately without the need to measure everything.
- **Listen to Your Hunger Cues:** Eat slowly and give your body time to signal when it's full. It takes about 20 minutes for the brain to recognize this signal, so pausing halfway through a meal can help prevent overeating.

The Advantages of Meal Prepping for Maintaining a Healthy Diet

Meal prepping involves preparing meals or ingredients ahead of time, providing a convenient way to stay on track with your weight loss goals. The advantages of this approach are numerous:

- **Saves Time and Reduces Stress:** Having meals ready to go or easy to assemble reduces daily decision-making and preparation time, making it easier to stick to a healthy diet.
- **Helps Manage Portions:** Pre-portioned meals ensure you consume just the right amount, aiding in calorie control.
- **Encourages Variety and Nutritional Balance:** Planning meals ahead allows for a variety of foods throughout the week, ensuring a balance of nutrients.
- **Avoids Unhealthy Eating Choices:** With meals prepared in advance, you're less likely to resort to fast food or processed snacks when hungry.

Ideas for Balanced Meals that are Both Nutritious and Satisfying

Creating meals that are balanced, nutritious, and satisfying is key to a successful weight loss plan. Here are ideas to inspire your meal planning:

Breakfast Ideas:

- **Greek Yogurt with Mixed Berries and a Sprinkle of Almonds:** Offers a blend of protein, healthy fats, and antioxidants.
- **Oatmeal Topped with Chia Seeds, Banana, and Cinnamon:** Provides a high-fiber start to the day, along with heart-healthy omega-3s from chia seeds.

Lunch Ideas:

- **Quinoa Salad with Chickpeas, Spinach, and Avocado:** A hearty, protein-packed salad that's rich in fiber and healthy fats.
- **Turkey and Avocado Wrap:** Using a whole grain tortilla, lean turkey, avocado, and plenty of vegetables for a satisfying and balanced meal.

Dinner Ideas:

- **Grilled Salmon with Steamed Broccoli and Quinoa:** Offers a perfect balance of omega-3 fatty acids, protein, and fiber.
- **Chicken Stir-fry with a Variety of Vegetables and Brown Rice:** A great way to incorporate multiple servings of vegetables with lean protein and whole grains.

Snack Ideas:

- **Vegetable Sticks with Hummus:** A crunchy, nutrient-rich snack that's also rich in protein and fiber.
- **A Small Handful of Nuts and a Piece of Fruit:** Provides a satisfying combination of healthy fats, protein, and fiber.

Conclusion

Planning your meals for weight loss is a multifaceted approach that extends beyond mere calorie counting. It encompasses mastering portion control, embracing the practice of meal prepping, and creating meals that are balanced and satisfying. This strategic approach not only supports your weight loss goals but also enriches your diet with a variety of nutrients essential for overall health. By implementing these strategies, you're more likely to enjoy a sustainable and enjoyable weight loss journey, ensuring that each meal is a step towards achieving your health and wellness goals.

Adopting healthy eating habits and practicing mindful eating are pivotal steps towards achieving and maintaining a healthy weight, especially when paired with a structured exercise program like chair yoga. These practices foster a deeper connection with food, allowing individuals to enjoy their meals fully while addressing the root causes of overeating and making healthier food choices consistently. This comprehensive approach to eating can transform one's relationship with food, leading to lasting weight loss and improved overall health.

Strategies for Adopting Mindful Eating Practices

Mindful eating is about being fully present for each eating experience, paying attention to the flavors, textures, and sensations of your food, and listening to your body's hunger and satiety signals. Here are effective strategies to incorporate mindful eating into your daily life:

- **Eat Without Distractions:** Sit at a table without the TV on, put away your phone, and focus solely on your meal. This helps you tune into your food and how it makes you feel.
- **Slow Down:** Take time to chew your food thoroughly and put down your utensil between bites. Slowing down can enhance digestion and make it easier to recognize when you're full.
- **Engage Your Senses:** Notice the smell, taste, and texture of your food. Appreciating these details can make meals more satisfying and help prevent overeating.
- **Check-In With Your Hunger:** Before eating, ask yourself how hungry you really are. Use a hunger scale of 1 to 10 to assess your hunger levels and decide how much food you really need.
- **Practice Gratitude for Your Food:** Take a moment before you begin eating to express gratitude for your meal. This can help you connect more deeply with the experience of eating.

Tips for Recognizing and Responding to True Hunger vs. Emotional Eating

Differentiating between true hunger and emotional eating is crucial for maintaining a healthy diet and preventing unnecessary weight gain. Here are tips to help you recognize and respond appropriately:

- **Identify Emotional Triggers:** Keep a food diary to note what you eat, when, and how you're feeling. Over time, you may notice patterns that indicate emotional eating, such as reaching for snacks when stressed or bored.
- **Find Non-Food Ways to Deal with Emotions:** If you identify that you're eating in response to emotions, find other ways to cope. This could be through exercise, meditation, talking with a friend, or engaging in a hobby.
- **Wait Before Eating:** When you feel an urge to eat driven by emotion rather than hunger, wait 10-15 minutes. Often, the craving will pass, indicating it was not true hunger.
- **Hydrate:** Sometimes, thirst is mistaken for hunger. Drink a glass of water and wait a few minutes to see if the hunger subsides.

How to Make Healthier Food Choices in Various Settings

Making healthier food choices consistently, regardless of the setting, is key to sustained weight loss and health. Whether you're at home, dining out, or attending social gatherings, here are strategies to ensure you stick to your health goals:

At Home:

- **Stock Up on Healthy Foods:** Keep your pantry and refrigerator filled with nutritious foods like fruits, vegetables, lean proteins, and whole grains. Having these foods readily available makes it easier to prepare healthy meals.
- **Plan Your Meals:** Use meal planning to ensure you have the ingredients for healthy meals throughout the week. This reduces the temptation to order takeout or eat processed foods.

In Restaurants:

- **Preview the Menu:** Look at the menu online ahead of time to decide on a healthy option without the pressure of the moment.
- **Ask for Modifications:** Don't hesitate to ask for dishes to be prepared in a healthier manner, such as grilled instead of fried or with the sauce on the side.
- **Be Mindful of Portions:** Restaurant portions can be large. Consider sharing a dish or asking for half to be boxed up before you start eating.

At Social Gatherings:

- **Eat Before You Go:** Having a small, healthy snack before attending a social event can prevent overindulgence.
- **Bring a Healthy Dish:** If it's a potluck, bring a dish that you know is healthy and satisfying. This ensures there's at least one nutritious option you can enjoy.
- **Focus on Socializing:** Make the event about connecting with others rather than the food. Engaging in conversation can distract from mindless eating.

Incorporating these mindful eating practices and strategies for making healthier food choices into your lifestyle can significantly impact your weight loss journey and overall health. By becoming more attuned to your body's hunger signals and emotional needs, you can develop a more balanced and satisfying relationship with food. Whether you're navigating daily meals at home or the challenges of eating out and socializing, these principles can guide you towards lasting health and wellness.

In the quest for weight loss and optimal health, the term "superfoods" frequently emerges, promising a plethora of health benefits thanks to their dense nutritional profiles. Understanding what constitutes a superfood, recognizing their benefits, particularly in relation to weight loss, and finding innovative ways to integrate them into your diet can significantly enhance your nutritional intake and support your weight loss journey.

Definition and Examples of Superfoods

Superfoods don't have a strict scientific definition but are generally recognized as foods that are rich in nutrients and antioxidants, offering health benefits beyond those of standard nutrients. These foods are prized for their high vitamins, minerals, fiber, antioxidant, and phytonutrient content, which can help fight chronic diseases, improve energy levels, and enhance overall health.

Examples of widely recognized superfoods include:

- **Berries (blueberries, strawberries, goji berries):** Packed with vitamins, fiber, and particularly high levels of antioxidants.
- **Leafy Greens (kale, spinach, Swiss chard):** High in vitamins A, C, E, K, and several B vitamins, as well as rich in antioxidants and fiber.
- **Nuts and Seeds (chia seeds, flaxseeds, almonds):** Excellent sources of healthy fats, protein, and fiber.
- **Whole Grains (quinoa, oats, barley):** Rich in fiber and protein, offering sustained energy and promoting digestive health.
- **Legumes (beans, lentils, chickpeas):** High in protein, fiber, and various nutrients while being low in fat.
- **Fatty Fish (salmon, mackerel, sardines):** Great sources of omega-3 fatty acids, known for their anti-inflammatory properties.

The Nutritional Benefits of Superfoods and Their Impact on Weight Loss

Superfoods can play a crucial role in weight loss due to their nutrient density and low calorie content. Incorporating these foods into your diet can offer several weight loss benefits:

- **High Fiber Content:** Many superfoods are high in fiber, which slows digestion and helps you feel fuller longer, reducing overall calorie intake.
- **Antioxidant Properties:** The antioxidants found in superfoods can help combat inflammation in the body, which is often linked to obesity and metabolic diseases.

- **Healthy Fats:** Foods like nuts, seeds, and fatty fish provide omega-3 fatty acids, which can enhance satiety and prevent snacking on unhealthy options.
- **Metabolism Boost:** Certain superfoods, such as green tea, contain compounds that can increase metabolic rate and fat burning.

Creative Ways to Incorporate Superfoods into the Diet

Integrating superfoods into your diet doesn't have to be complicated or bland. Here are some creative and delicious ways to enjoy these nutrient-packed foods:

Start with Smoothies

Smoothies are a fantastic way to pack several superfoods into one delicious and convenient meal or snack. Blend leafy greens like spinach or kale with berries, a banana for sweetness, and a tablespoon of chia or flaxseeds for a nutrient-rich drink.

Upgrade Your Salads

Turn a simple salad into a superfood feast by incorporating a variety of colorful vegetables, a handful of nuts for crunch, and a serving of quinoa or chickpeas for added protein and fiber. Dress with a simple vinaigrette made with extra virgin olive oil (another superfood) and lemon juice.

Snack Smart

Swap out processed snacks for superfood alternatives. Almonds, walnuts, or pumpkin seeds make for satisfying, nutrient-dense snacks. Berries or sliced apple with almond butter offer a sweet yet healthy treat.

Supercharge Your Soups and Stews

Add lentils, beans, or chickpeas to soups and stews to boost their nutritional profile. Leafy greens like kale or Swiss chard can also be easily incorporated into these dishes in the last few minutes of cooking, adding vitamins and minerals without compromising taste.

Make Superfood Breakfasts

Start your day with a superfood boost by adding oats, quinoa, or chia seeds to your breakfast. Top with berries, nuts, and a drizzle of honey for a balanced meal. Alternatively, eggs (considered by many as a superfood) scrambled with spinach, tomatoes, and mushrooms can provide a protein-rich start to the day.

In conclusion, superfoods are more than just a trend; they're a powerful component of a balanced diet that can significantly support weight loss and overall health. By incorporating a variety of these nutrient-dense foods into your meals, you not only enhance the flavor and diversity of your diet but also supply your body with the essential nutrients it needs to function optimally, manage weight, and combat disease. With creativity and a bit of planning, making superfoods a regular part of your eating habits can be both enjoyable and incredibly beneficial.

REVOLUTIONIZE YOUR BODY IN 28 DAYS

	Exercise
Day 1	• Seated Calf Raises • Seated Ankle Circles • Seated Jacks • Seated Mountain Pose with Deep Breathing • Seated Scapular Retraction
Day 2	• Chair Marching with Arm Swings • Seated Side Leg Raises • Seated Knee Extensions • Chair Spinal Twist • Seated Leg Extensions with Arm Raises
Day 3	• Seated Side Steps • Chair Extended Side Angle • Chair Eagle Arms • Seated Leg Lifts • Chair Arm Raises
Day 4	• Seated Arm Twists • Seated Hip Openers

	• Seated Eagle Arms • Seated Shoulder Circles • Chair Savasana
Day 5	• Chair Tap Dancing • Seated Cat-Cow Stretch • Chair Pigeon Pose • Seated Marching Hip Lifts • Seated Leg Cross
Day 6	• Chair Marching • Chair Pigeon Pose • Seated Forward Bend • Chair Warrior II • Seated Twist
Day 7	• Chair Eagle Arms • Seated Mountain Pose with Deep Breathing • Seated Calf Raises • Seated Shoulder Circles • Seated Hip Openers
Day 8	• Seated Leg Extensions with Arm Raises • Seated Eagle Arms

	• Seated Knee Extensions • Seated Cat-Cow Stretch • Seated Side Leg Raises
Day 9	• Chair Extended Side Angle • Chair Savasana • Chair Arm Raises • Seated Marching Hip Lifts • Seated Twist
Day 10	• Chair Spinal Twist • Chair Pigeon Pose • Seated Ankle Circles • Seated Side Steps • Seated Leg Cross
Day 11	• Seated Arm Twists • Seated Jacks • Chair Warrior II • Chair Marching • Chair Tap Dancing
Day 12	• Seated Leg Lifts • Seated Forward Bend

	• Chair Pigeon Pose • Chair Marching with Arm Swings • Seated Scapular Retraction
Day 13	• Seated Scapular Retraction • Seated Jacks • Seated Ankle Circles • Chair Savasana • Chair Pigeon Pose
Day 14	• Chair Spinal Twist • Seated Twist • Chair Eagle Arms • Seated Cat-Cow Stretch • Seated Mountain Pose with Deep Breathing
Day 15	• Chair Pigeon Pose • Seated Knee Extensions • Seated Calf Raises • Chair Tap Dancing • Seated Marching Hip Lifts
Day 16	• Seated Forward Bend • Seated Hip Openers

	• Seated Leg Cross • Chair Arm Raises • Chair Marching with Arm Swings
Day 17	• Seated Side Steps • Seated Leg Lifts • Seated Shoulder Circles • Chair Warrior II • Seated Arm Twists
Day 18	• Seated Eagle Arms • Seated Leg Extensions with Arm Raises • Chair Extended Side Angle • Seated Side Leg Raises • Chair Marching
Day 19	• Seated Marching Hip Lifts • Chair Extended Side Angle • Chair Marching with Arm Swings • Seated Mountain Pose with Deep Breathing • Seated Side Leg Raises
Day 20	• Chair Pigeon Pose • Seated Knee Extensions

	<ul><li>Seated Calf Raises</li><li>Seated Eagle Arms</li><li>Seated Jacks</li></ul>
Day 21	<ul><li>Chair Tap Dancing</li><li>Seated Scapular Retraction</li><li>Seated Ankle Circles</li><li>Chair Warrior II</li><li>Seated Side Steps</li></ul>
Day 22	<ul><li>Chair Spinal Twist</li><li>Chair Marching</li><li>Chair Arm Raises</li><li>Seated Hip Openers</li><li>Seated Cat-Cow Stretch</li></ul>
Day 23	<ul><li>Chair Savasana</li><li>Chair Pigeon Pose</li><li>Seated Leg Cross</li><li>Seated Leg Lifts</li><li>Seated Twist</li></ul>
Day 24	<ul><li>Chair Eagle Arms</li><li>Seated Forward Bend</li></ul>

	• Seated Shoulder Circles • Seated Arm Twists • Seated Leg Extensions with Arm Raises
Day 25	• Chair Savasana • Chair Marching • Seated Eagle Arms • Seated Leg Lifts • Seated Jacks
Day 26	• Seated Side Leg Raises • Seated Mountain Pose with Deep Breathing • Chair Pigeon Pose • Seated Twist • Seated Shoulder Circles
Day 27	• Chair Warrior II • Seated Leg Extensions with Arm Raises • Chair Spinal Twist • Seated Calf Raises • Chair Pigeon Pose
Day 28	• Seated Forward Bend • Chair Extended Side Angle

<table>
<tr><td></td><td>

- Seated Arm Twists

- Chair Eagle Arms

- Seated Ankle Circles

</td></tr>
</table>

CONCLUSION

As we draw the curtains on this comprehensive exploration of Chair Yoga and its multifaceted benefits for seniors, let's reflect on the journey we've undertaken. Through the various chapters, we've delved into the fundamentals of Chair Yoga, breathing and meditation techniques, the significance of these exercises for weight loss, and the overarching benefits they present for daily activities. This conclusion aims to weave together the insights and knowledge shared, emphasizing the transformative power of Chair Yoga for enhancing senior health and well-being.

Embracing Chair Yoga: A Path to Enhanced Well-being

Chair Yoga emerges as a beacon of accessibility and inclusivity within the yoga practice, tailored to meet the needs and limitations of seniors and individuals with mobility issues. This gentle form of yoga, utilizing a chair for support, opens the door to the myriad benefits of yoga practice, traditionally accessible only to those able to engage in more physically demanding poses. The beauty of Chair Yoga lies in its adaptability, offering modifications that cater to various fitness levels, ensuring everyone can partake in the journey towards health and vitality.

The Symphony of Breathing and Meditation

Breathing and meditation, the pillars of yoga practice, have been highlighted for their profound impact on mental and emotional well-being. These practices invite a sense of calm and clarity, serving as powerful tools for managing stress, enhancing cognitive function, and fostering an inner peace that transcends the yoga mat. For seniors, the integration of these practices into daily life can be particularly transformative, offering strategies to navigate the challenges of aging with grace and resilience.

Weight Loss and Beyond: The Holistic Benefits of Chair Yoga

The exploration of Chair Yoga's efficacy in supporting weight loss underscores the holistic nature of yoga practice. Beyond the physical benefits of improved flexibility, strength, and balance, Chair Yoga contributes to metabolic health and cardiovascular well-being. It's a testament to the idea that health is not merely the absence of disease but a state of complete physical, mental, and social well-being. Chair

Yoga, with its gentle approach, provides a pathway to achieve this holistic health, making it particularly suited for seniors looking to maintain an active and fulfilling lifestyle.

Daily Activities Reimagined: The Practical Impact of Chair Yoga

Chair Yoga's influence extends into the realm of daily activities, offering seniors a renewed sense of independence and vitality. The exercises and techniques presented throughout this book are designed not just for the yoga session but for integration into everyday life. From enhancing mobility and stability to reducing the risk of falls, the benefits of Chair Yoga translate into a more active, confident, and autonomous existence for seniors.

The Community Aspect: Chair Yoga as a Social Catalyst

An often-overlooked benefit of Chair Yoga is its ability to foster community and connection among practitioners. Yoga classes, whether in-person or virtual, provide a sense of belonging and shared purpose, crucial elements for mental health and well-being. For seniors, this social interaction is invaluable, offering support, friendship, and a shared space for growth and healing.

Looking Ahead: Incorporating Chair Yoga into Your Life

As we conclude, the invitation is to incorporate Chair Yoga into your life, not as a temporary intervention but as a sustained practice. The journey of yoga is one of continuous exploration and discovery, with each practice session offering new insights into the body, mind, and spirit. By making Chair Yoga a regular part of your routine, you open yourself up to ongoing improvements in health, well-being, and quality of life.

Conclusion

This book has endeavored to present Chair Yoga as a comprehensive, accessible, and beneficial practice for seniors and individuals with mobility issues. From the physical benefits of improved strength and flexibility to the mental and emotional gains of stress reduction and enhanced cognitive function, Chair Yoga stands out as a holistic practice. It offers a pathway to health and vitality that respects the body's limitations while celebrating its capabilities.

As you move forward, remember that the practice of yoga is not about reaching the perfect pose but about finding balance, harmony, and contentment within oneself. Chair Yoga, with its adaptations and modifications, ensures that this journey is accessible to all, inviting practitioners to explore their potential and embrace a healthier, more vibrant life.

In the words of the ancient yoga sutras, "Yoga is the journey of the self, through the self, to the self." May your journey with Chair Yoga be filled with discovery, transformation, and profound well-being.